NATURAL
BODY CARE

More than 60 Simple
techniques to Enhance
Your Health & Beauty

SILVERLEAF
PRESS

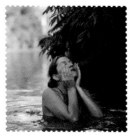

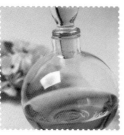

Contents

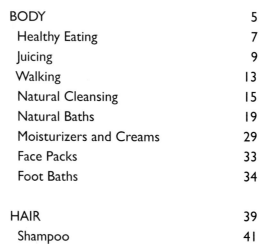

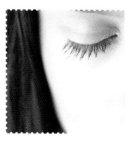

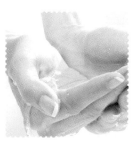

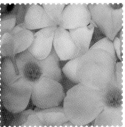

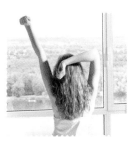

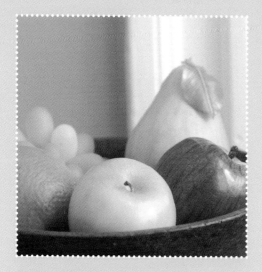
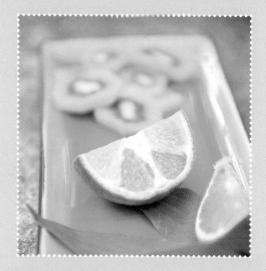
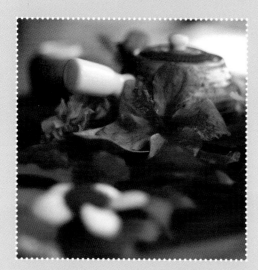
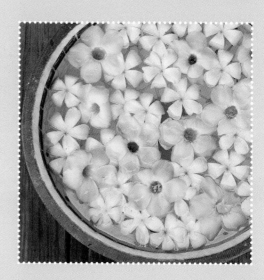

BODY

Enhance your daily life by learning to naturally care for your body from the inside out. Incorporate these simple ideas into your lifestyle and you will begin to look and feel your best in no time.

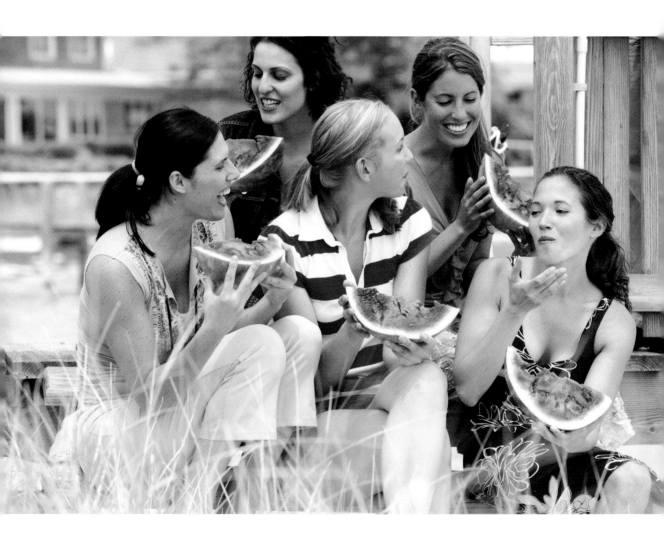

6

HEALTHY EATING

Making small changes to your diet will not only increase your energy levels but will also improve your overall health. Choose high protein foods rich in vitamins and minerals. Eat plenty of complex carbohydrates, fresh raw fruit and vegetables, and eat the right fats, such as olive oil and flax oil instead of margarine or butter. In a relatively short amount of time, you will notice a definite change in the way you feel.

High Energy Foods

Apples
✢ A great antioxidant and loaded with vitamin C
✢ Great for detoxing the body

Avocado
✢ High in polyunsaturated fat
✢ Keeps skin soft and boosts metabolism
✢ Lessens fatigue and keeps skin soft

Fresh nuts
(almonds, hazels, Brazils, pinola, and chestnuts)
✢ High in protein
✢ Lessens fatigue and keeps skin soft

Garlic
✢ Boosts cell renewal

Kiwi Fruit
✢ Loaded with vitamins C and E and potassium
✢ Great for moods and digestion

Lemon
✢ Helps thin the blood and clean the liver

Carrots
✢ High in beta-carotene
✢ Supports a healthy liver

Oily Fish
(salmon, herring, mackerel)
✢ Contains essential fatty acids
✢ Fights fatigue and boosts circulation

Sesame seeds
✢ Helps support a healthy liver and kidneys

Yogurt
✢ High in vitamin B, zinc, and potassium
✢ Great for detoxing the body, promotes gastrointestinal health, and aids in the absorption of vitamin B

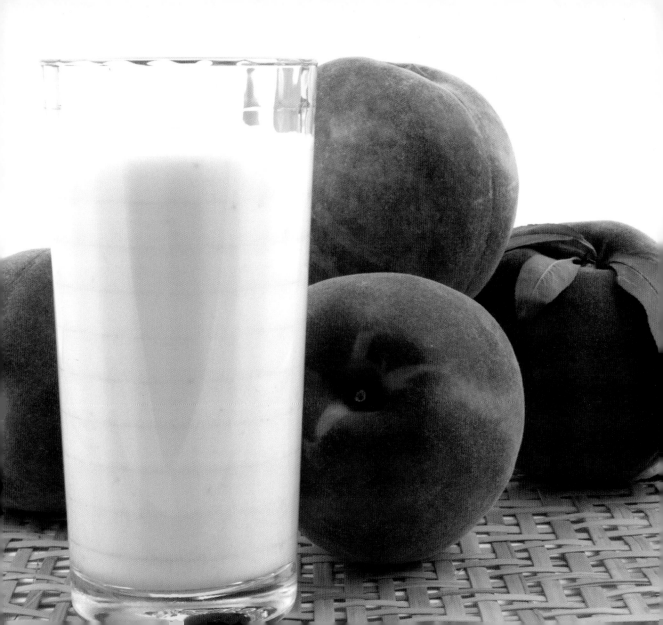

JUICING

Juicing is a great way to increase your strength, energy, and overall good health. Juicing gives you a natural concentrated source of vitamins, minerals, and enzymes. These naturally occurring supplements will give you a lasting, powerful nutrition boost. Below is a list of the best food sources for vitamins and minerals. As you get better at juicing, you can create your own recipes using the fruits and vegetables that are suited to your specific needs.

Fruit is packed with nutrients, but also contains a high quantity of natural sugars. It is recommended that our intake of pure fruit juice should not exceed 8 ounces a day. Instead, fruit juice can be added to vegetable juices for a natural sweetness.

To Begin

✤ You need to begin the juicing process with a good juicer that has a strong motor (½ horsepower or more).

✤ Keep your juicer in an easily accessible place where it will be convenient to use every day.

✤ Use organic fruits and vegetables. Wash them thoroughly to remove any dirt. If you decide to use conventionally grown produce, peel them; the peels are more likely to contain pesticides.

✤ Wash, peel, and cut fruits and veggies in advance and store them, covered, in the refrigerator.

The Basic Cocktail

3 medium carrots, green tops removed

2 stalks celery

1 1-inch piece ginger root

½ low-sugar apple (Granny Smith or Pippin)

Carrot-Apple Juice

6 medium carrots, green tops removed

2 Golden Delicious apples

The Pick-Me-Up

4 medium carrots

3 fennel stalks with leaves and flowers

1 stalk organic celery with leaves

½ small or medium lemon

Vitamins

B1
✤ supports energy metabolism and nerve function
✤ spinach, green peas, tomatoes, watermelon

B2
✤ supports energy metabolism, normal vision and skin health
✤ spinach, broccoli, mushrooms

B3
✤ supports energy metabolism, skin health, nervous system and digestive system
✤ spinach, potatoes, tomatoes

B6
✤ aids amino acid and fatty acid metabolism and red blood cell production
✤ bananas, watermelon, tomatoes, broccoli, spinach, acorn squash, potatoes
✤ great for moods and digestion

FOLATE
✤ supports DNA synthesis and new cell formation
✤ tomatoes, green beans, broccoli, spinach, asparagus

C
✤ aids collagen synthesis, amino acid metabolism, helps iron absorption and immunity, acts as an antioxidant
✤ spinach, broccoli, red bell peppers, snow peas, tomatoes, kiwi, mango, oranges, grapefruit, strawberries

A
✤ supports vision, skin, bones, and tooth growth, immunity, and reproduction
✤ mango, broccoli, butternut squash, carrots, tomatoes, sweet potatoes, pumpkin

E
✤ acts as an antioxidant, aids in regulation of oxidation reactions, supports cell membrane stabilization
✤ avocado, sweet potatoes

K
✤ synthesis of blood-clotting proteins, regulates blood calcium
✤ Brussel sprouts, leafy green vegetables, spinach, broccoli, cabbage

Minerals

POTASSIUM
✤ maintains fluid and electrolyte balance, cell integrity, muscle contractions and nerve impulse transmission
✤ potatoes, acorn squash, artichoke, spinach, broccoli, carrots, green beans, tomatoes, avocado, grapefruit, watermelon, banana, strawberries, spinach, green peas, tomatoes, watermelon

ZINC
✤ a part of many enzymes, involved in production of genetic material and proteins, transports vitamin A, improves taste perception and healing wounds, aids sperm production and the normal development of the fetus
✤ spinach, broccoli, green peas, green beans, tomatoes

MAGNESIUM
✤ supports bone mineralization, aids in protein building, muscular contraction, nerve impulse transmission, and immunity
✤ spinach, broccoli, artichokes, green beans, tomatoes

IRON
✤ part of the protein hemoglobin (carries oxygen throughout body's cells)
✤ artichokes, parsley, spinach, broccoli, green beans, tomatoes

CALCIUM
✤ aids in formation of bones and teeth, and in blood clotting
✤ green beans, spinach, broccoli

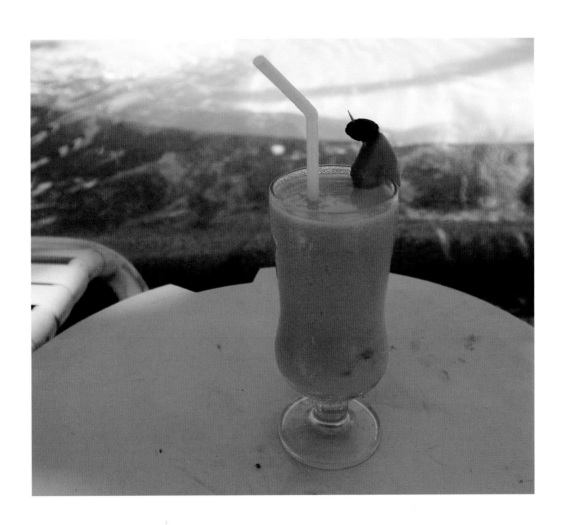

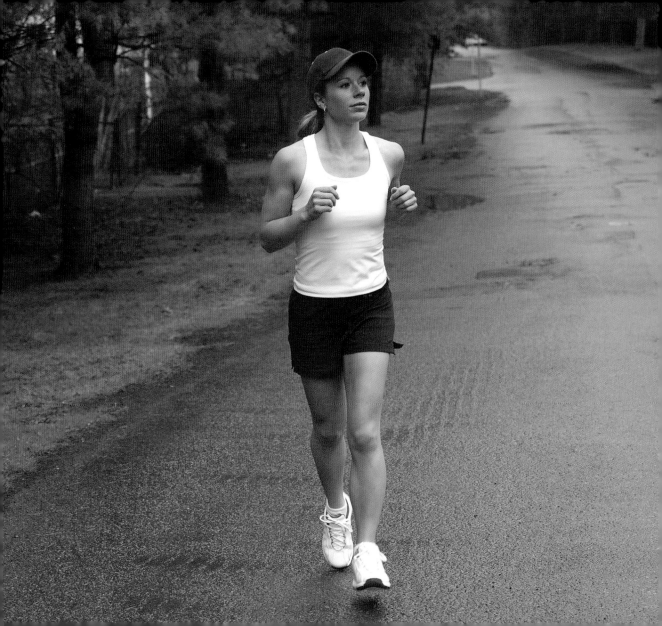

WALKING

Walking is one of the easiest and most effective ways of getting in shape—and staying that way. It is a fantastic way to burn calories while providing your cardio system and muscles with a great workout. Walking is also a way to reduce stress and produce invigorating energy; help with diabetes, osteoporosis, back pain, and a variety of other health problems. Done consistently and correctly, walking can tone your body and boost your metabolism.

While you can walk practically anywhere, you need to vary the terrain, duration, and intensity of your routine if you want to lose weight. For overall better health, stride at a steady pace and breathe easily for at least 30 minutes a day. Follow these simple guidelines to reap the benefits of the world's simplest exercise.

To Begin

1. Hold head erect, keep your back straight and stomach flat. Make sure your toes are pointing straight ahead.
2. Hit your heel to the ground first and roll off the ball of your foot, making sure you don't lock your knees.
3. Transfer your weight onto the other foot, hitting your heel to the ground first, and take your next step.
4. Take deep breaths through your nose or mouth, whichever is most comfortable.
5. Drive your elbows forward and back as you take each step, keeping your hips and shoulders squared.

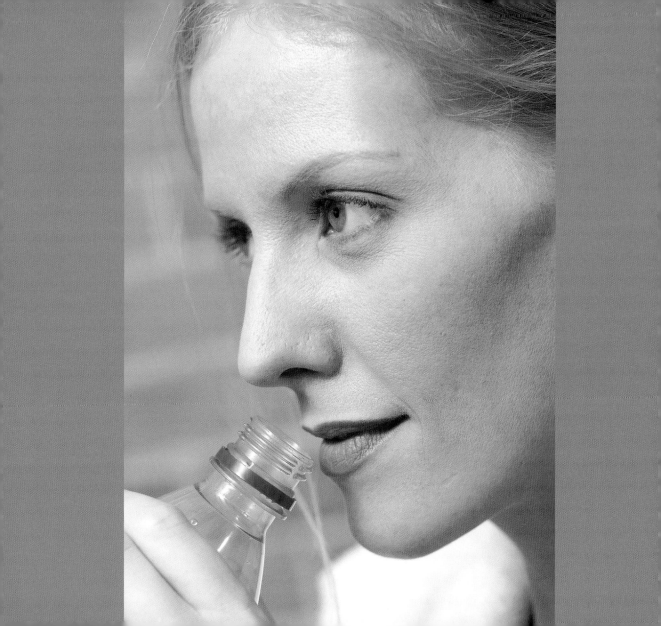

NATURAL CLEANSING

Herbal Detox

An essential part of good health is detoxification. We live in an environment where toxins are present in the air we breathe, the foods we eat, and the water we drink. Our bodies are over-stressed with the accumulation of toxins that are detrimental to our health. Removal of these toxins will help you feel restored, energized, and refreshed.

Herbs work wonders for detoxification purposes as they stimulate the liver, lungs, and kidneys maximizing their ability to cleanse. But it is important to use them in conjunction with a good diet. Below is a list of herbal combinations and the organs they benefit.

Herbal Combinations

Liver
dandelion, red beet, liverwort, parsley, horsetail, birch leaves, chamomile, blessed thistle, black cohosh, angelica, gentian, goldenrod

Kidneys
parsley, dandelion, juniper berries, marshmallow, ginger, goldenseal, dong quai, cedar berries

Lungs
comfrey, marshmallow, mullein, slippery elm, senega, Chinese ephedra

How to Herbal Cleanse

Morning
1 teaspoon apple cider vinegar
1 teaspoon blackstrap molasses
OR
2 slices lemon

Mix 8 ounces glass pure water with 1 teaspoon apple cider vinegar and 1 teaspoon blackstrap molasses or 2 lemon slices.

Mid-morning
2 teaspoons psyllium husk powder
8 ounces glass pure water

Mix and drink. Follow with another glass pure water.

In Between/Mealtimes
Take 2–3 multi-digestive enzymes and liver herbs at mealtimes and drink herbal tea, which supports the liver, between meals.

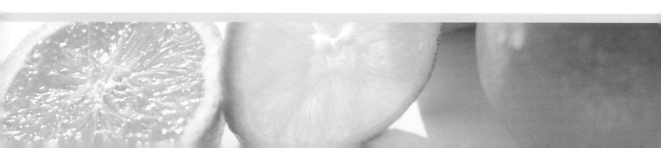

Skin Cleansing

Skin is an eliminative organ; therefore our detoxification routine should include some type of skin cleansing. Toxins are released through the pores of the skin when we sweat. Using saunas and steam rooms are a fantastic way to remove the harmful toxins.

Daily bathing using natural soaps and shampoos is another way to cleanse the skin. Toweling roughly after, until the skin is slightly red, is a great way to remove the outer dead skin layers and open the pores. Be sure to change towels often.

Detox Bath

Try this relaxing bath once a month to remove aluminum and mercury from your system. Use it once a week during a detoxification routine.

Place ½ cup baking soda, ½ cup Epsom salt, or ½ cup sea salt to a tub of warm water. Soak for 15–20 minutes. Scrub the skin gently using a natural soap and cotton cloth.

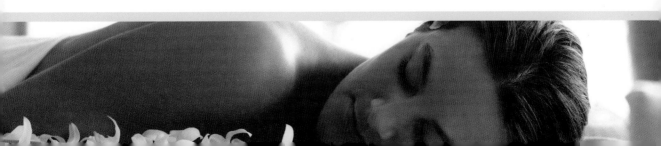

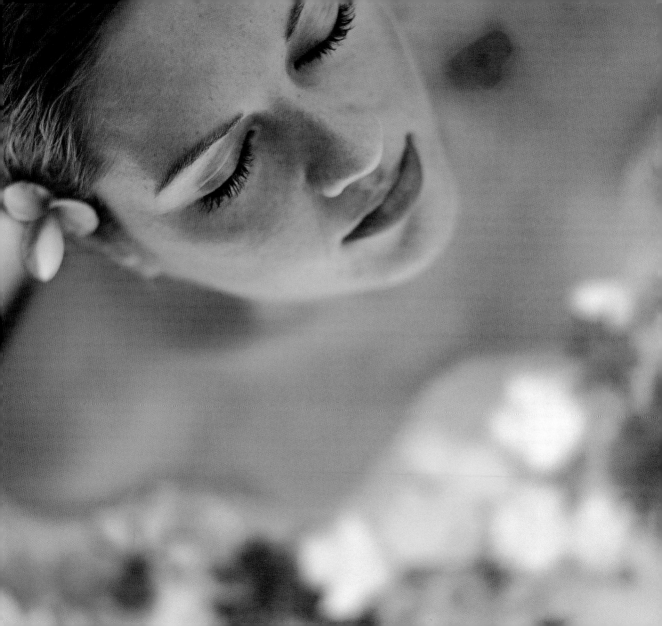

NATURAL BATHS

Herbal Baths

There is nothing like the pleasure of a long soak in a warm bath when tension and tiredness are making us feel wretched; we emerge from the water soothed and revived. Herbs can add to our pleasure and recovery for they have properties which, released into the water; can smooth and soothe the skin, deodorize, relax the nerves or stimulate flagging energy.

BATH HERBS

Stimulating
✤ basil, bay, fennel, lavender, lemon verbena, lovage, meadowsweet, mint, pine, rosemary, sage, thyme

Healing
✤ comfrey, lady's mantle, marigold, mint, yarrow

Relaxing
✤ catmint, chamomile, jasmine, lime flowers, vervain

Relieving fatigue and aching limbs
✤ bay, bergamot, mugwort, rosemary

Herbal Bath Bags

You can also put a handful of herbs into a little muslin bag and hang the bag by a long loop to the hot tap so that the water will flow through the bag as the bath is run.

Make it a long loop so that the bag is under the water as quickly as possible—the heat of the water will release the properties of the herbs and they will be lost in the steam if the bag is left in the air.

Herbal Bath Infusion

Infusions need to be concentrated as they are mixed with a large volume of water.

2 ounces (50g) dried or 4 ounces (100g) of fresh herbs
1 pint (475mL) boiling water
jug
sieve

1. Put the herbs of your choice into the jug. Add the boiling water and leave to infuse for 30 minutes.
2. Strain the infusion through the sieve and add to the bath water.

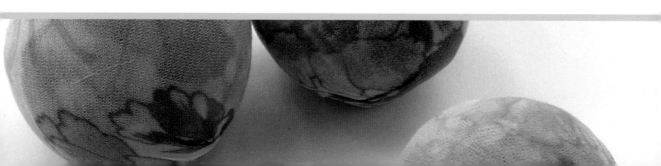

Herbal Bath Decoction

This mixture contains bran to soften the water.

4 ounces (100g) fresh herbs
1 ounces (25g) bran
1½ pints (700mL) boiling water
stainless steel saucepan
sieve

1. Put herbs in saucepan, add water and gently bring to boil. Keep simmering until the color of the water is quite strong. About 30 minutes.
2. Strain the mixture through the sieve and add to the bath water.

A Tonic Bath

A tonic bath is good when the skin looks dingy and tired.

6 ounces (170g) young blackberry shoots and leaves
2⅓ cups (545mL) of water
saucepan
sieve

1. Combine water and blackberry leaves in saucepan and heat to 115°F (45°C).
2. Infuse for about 5 minutes, strain through sieve and add to the warm bath.

Similar tonics can be made using nettle, dandelion, or daisies. Allow 1 pound (450g) of dried plant to every 8 pints (4L) of water. Allow the flowers or herbs to steep in the water for about 30 minutes. Then strain and add to the warm bath.

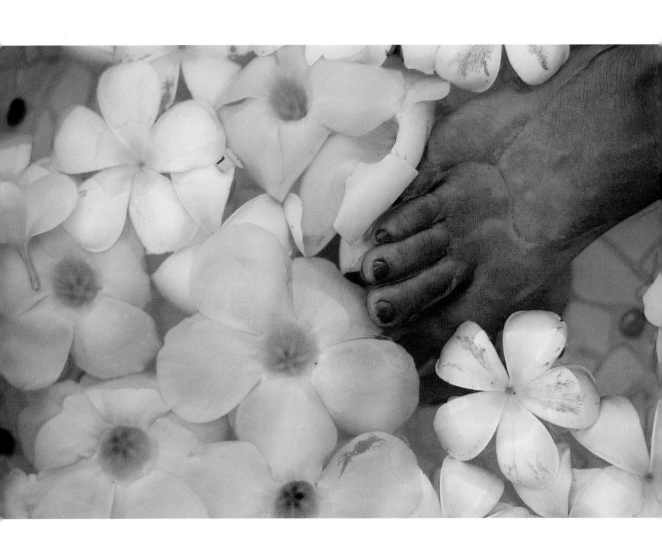

✿ NATURAL BODY CARE ✿

Skin-smoothing Vinegar Bath

A vinegar bath soothes itchiness and aching muscles and softens the skin and the bath water. The following is enough for two baths.

1/2 pint (240mL) cider vinegar
1/2 pint (240mL) spring water
1 ounces (25g) dried herbs or 2 ounces (50g) fresh herbs
stainless steel saucepan
bowl with cover
sieve bottle

1. Put the cider vinegar, spring water and selected herbs into the saucepan. Heat to simmering, but do not boil.
2. Pour the mixture into a bowl and cover. Leave for 12 hours then strain and bottle.

After-bath Cologne

Use this fragrant cologne as a friction rub after a bath.

½ cup (120mL) any strong scented fresh flower petals (rose, jasmine, carnation, etc.)
½ cup (120mL) deodorized alcohol or food grade isopropyl alcohol (can be obtained from most chemists)
1½ cups (350mL) very hot water
3 tablespoons ground citrus peel
1 tablespoon dried basil or lemon verbena
1 tablespoon mint or crushed thyme
cheesecloth or muslin

1. Soak flowers in the alcohol for one week in a tightly closed jar. On the sixth day, make an infusion of the peel and herbs in the hot water. Allow to stand for 24 hours.
2. Strain through cheesecloth or muslin. Drain petals. Combine the two liquids in a bottle with a screw top and shake well.

HERBAL PROPERTIES

Deodorant herbs

✤ basil and lovage

Tonic herbs

✤ Balm, basil, bergamot, pennyroyal, rosemary, sage

Astringent herbs

✤ Balm (gentle), chamomile (gentle), chervil (gentle), fennel (gentle), parsley (gentle), plantain, rosemary sage (strong), witch hazel, yarrow (strong)

Cleansing herbs

✤ Borage, chamomile, dandelion, elderflower, lime, lovage, nettle, plantain

Healing herbs

✤ Comfrey, lady's mantle, marigold, marshmallow, mint

Antiseptic herbs

✤ Lavender, mint, thyme, witch hazel

Soothing herbs

✤ Balm, burdock, chamomile, coltsfoot, comfrey, elderflower, lime flowers, marigold
✤ To relieve tension: chamomile, lemon, verbena, lime flowers, marjoram, meadowsweet, rosemary, and valerian
✤ To ease aching limbs: bay, bergamot, hyssop, marjoram, mugwort, rosemary
✤ To ease a bruised body: comfrey root and mint used together

Cosmetic herbs

✤ For oily skin: marigold flowers, horsetail, sage, and yarrow
✤ For dry skin: borage, lady's mantle, marshmallow, parsley, sorrel, and violet
✤ For aging skin: dandelion, elderflower, tansy, and verbena

Herbal Washers

To add to the effect of the bath, use this washer; pressing the bag against your body to cleanse and soften the skin. Stroke arms, legs, and back rhythmically and slowly.

4 tablespoons dried herbs of your choice
2 tablespoons oatmeal for cleansing (or 2 tbsp whole powdered milk, in place of oatmeal, if you wish to soften the skin)
a muslin bag

1. Combine a handful of herbs of your choice with a handful of fine oatmeal.
2. Place into a muslin bag—roll it up tightly or sew it up and use as a washer.

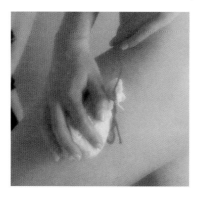

Steam Baths

The purpose of the steam bath is to bring out deep-seated impurities and to improve the complexion by stimulating circulation. It is far more suitable for an open-pored thick oily skin than for a thin sensitive one or one with evident thread-veins. It is fairly drastic treatment.

1. Put 1 tablespoon of dried chamomile, lime, or elder flowers in a bowl and pour ½ pint (240mL) boiling water over them.
2. Lean over the steam which is rising and drape a towel over your head and the bowl to contain the hot vapor.
3. Don't let the steam blast directly on to your face—keep it more than 12 inches (30cm) away. Close your eyes and keep still while the hot steam opens the pores and the properties in the herbs released into the steam by the hot water take effect. This should not last longer than 10 minutes. Remove towel and blot face dry.
4. Splash the face with cool water to close the pores. And stay indoors for a time if the weather is cold. The skin will be soft, pink, and clean-looking. If it feels tight, wipe it over, very gently, with moisturizer.

*Note: Chamomile flowers seem to please most people—comfrey, horsetail, nettle, rosemary, elderflower and lime flowers, peppermint, lady's mantle and yarrow are also used.

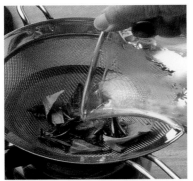

CHOOSING HERBS FOR A STEAM BATH

For an oily skin
horsetail, marigold flowers, sage, yarrow

For a dry skin
borage, lady's mantle, marshmallow, parsley, sorrel, violet

For an aging skin
dandelion, elderflower, red clover, tansy, verbena

MOISTURIZERS AND CREAMS

This mixture contains bran to soften the water.

Herbal Moisturizer

1. Soak some fresh or dried chamomile, lime, or elder flowers in full-cream milk overnight.
2. Strain, warm, and add a little honey to the liquid and use when the honey has dissolved. Keep the remainder in a sealed bottle in the refrigerator and use before the milk begins to go off.

Soothing Cream

1 tablespoon dried chamomile or elder flowers
almond or sunflower oil (enough to cover the herbs)
2 teaspoons lanolin
1 teaspoon honey

1. Put flowers in a jam jar and cover with the oil.
2. Melt lanolin and pour over the mixture. Place jar on a plate in a slow oven and leave for 20 minutes or stand the jar on an upturned saucer in a saucepan containing enough hot water to come partway up the jar and keep the water simmering gently.
3. Strain, then add the honey. Stir well. Pot when cool.

Daytime Moisturizing Cream

1 teaspoon each beeswax, lanolin and almond (or other) oil
1 capsule vitamin E oil
3 teaspoons rosewater
touch of borax

1. Melt beeswax and lanolin and stir well to combine.
2. Add warm oils gradually and beat well. Dissolve borax in warmed rosewater and beat into the mixture. Beat until cool and thickened. You can add a few drops of your favorite essential oil to give fragrance. Pot in a pretty jar.

Marigold Cream

1 cup (240mL) strong marigold petal tea
equal quantities beeswax, lanolin and almond, sunflower or wheat germ oil—about 2 teaspoons each
touch of borax powder

1. Dissolve wax, lanolin, and oil and mix together. Dissolve borax in the warm tea. Working slowly and carefully, gradually pour some of each mixture into a bowl, beating and mixing as you go.
2. Continue until all ingredients are used. Keep on beating and mixing until the mixture thickens and cools.

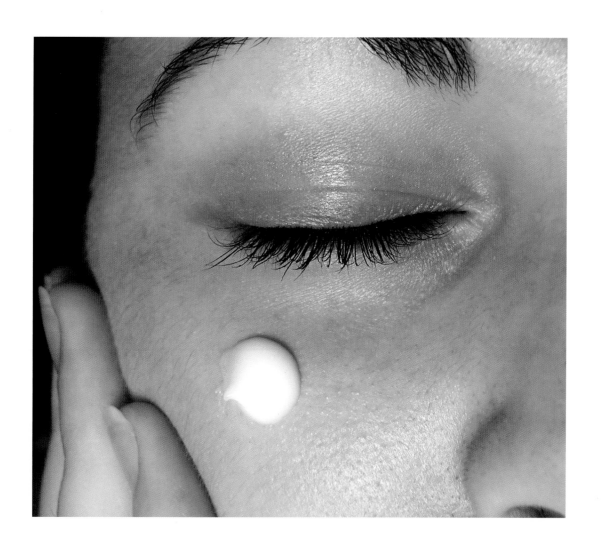

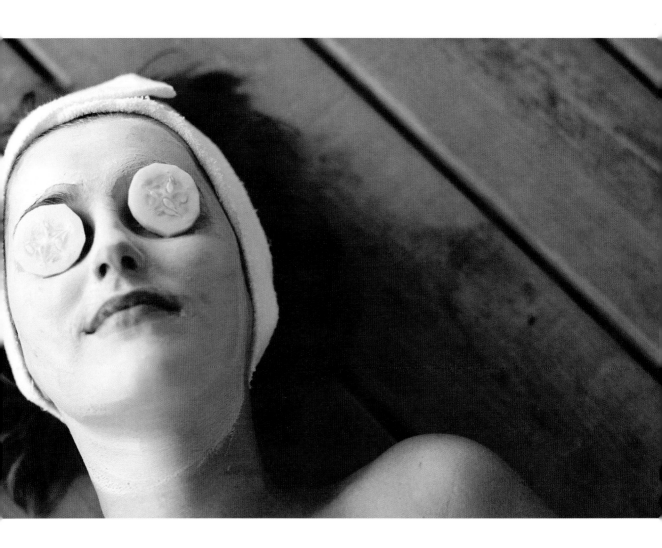

❀ NATURAL BODY CARE ❀

FACE PACKS

Face packs draw out impurities and stimulate the circulation. They suit thick oily skins better than thin dry ones.

The basis for a face pack can be fuller's earth, fine oatmeal, or ground almonds, if you are feeling flush. Fuller's earth looks like mud, oatmeal like porridge.

Face Pack For Oily Skin

1. Make a cup of strong yarrow tea and allow to cool.
2. Beat up an egg white. Mix the two ingredients with enough fine oatmeal to make a paste and add a touch of cider vinegar.
3. Apply the paste to the face for no more than half an hour keeping it away from the eyes. Lie down while the paste dries. Wash the paste off with tepid water.

Face Pack For Dry Skin

1. Make a paste from fine oatmeal, a little tea made from marigold petals, a little honey, some almond, sunflower, or wheat germ oil, and a beaten egg yolk.
2. Add a touch of cider vinegar and mix well. Use as described above.

FOOTBATHS

Herbal Foot Bath

Bathing the feet is a time-honored restorative. A mustard footbath will warm the whole body—a footbath containing herbs will ease it. Horsetail is excellent for tired feet and if used regularly will reduce perspiration. Lovage is a good deodorant—lavender, sage, peppermint, and thyme are instant refreshing tonics. Marjoram is soothing.

2 ounces (50g) herbs
1½ pints (700mL) water
saucepan
sieve
2 tablespoons sea salt

1. Boil herbs and water in a saucepan. Simmer for 30 minutes. Strain and stir in sea salt to make a decoction.
2. Add ½ pint (240mL) of the decoction to a bowl of hot water. Soak feet for 10 minutes.

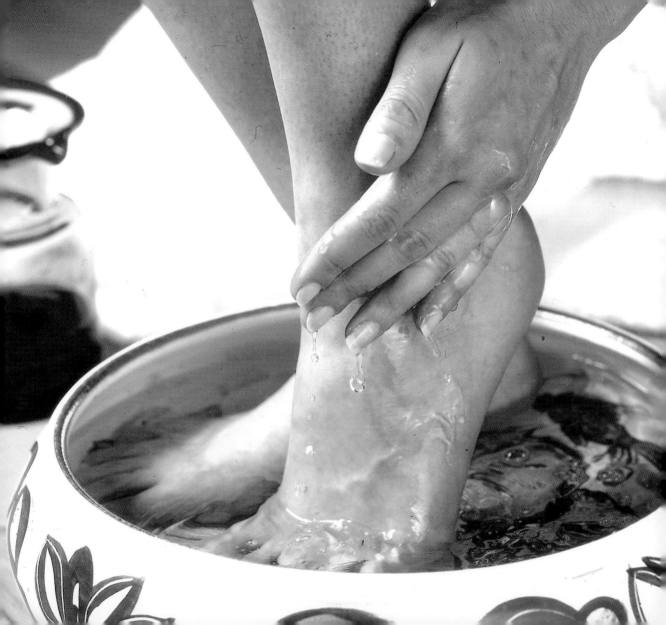

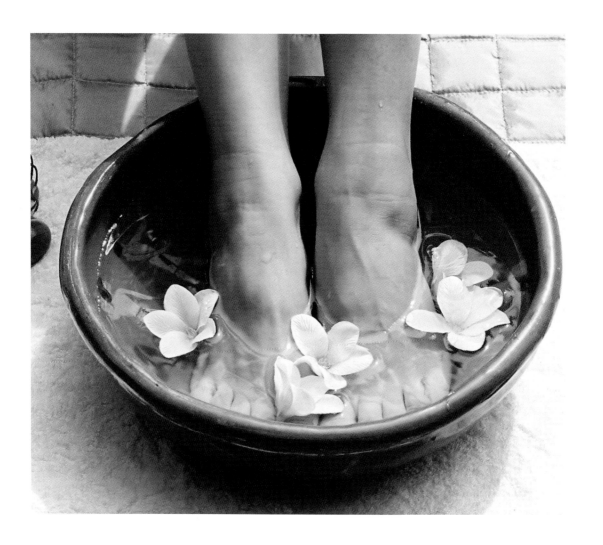

✿ NATURAL BODY CARE ✿

Lemonade Foot Soak

The acidity of the fruit will wash away dirt, grime, and dead skin cells. This lemon soak will soften your aching, tired feet and the aroma will cool you down and awaken your senses.

1 gallon (3.8L) fresh lemonade, warmed
2 drops lemon essential oil
4 lemons, sliced
1 lemon, halved
¼ cup granulated sugar

Pour the lemonade into a large tub. Add the oil and slices, and soak your feet for 2 minutes. Dip the lemon halves in the sugar and scrub away any rough skin. Rinse with warm water.

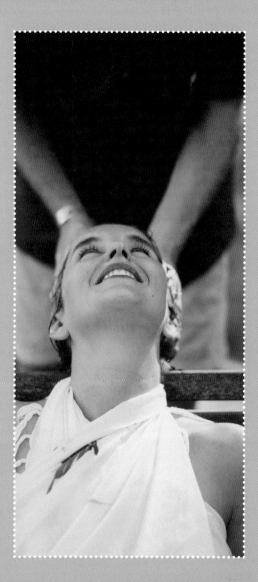
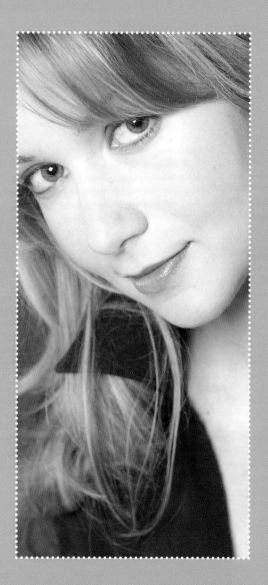

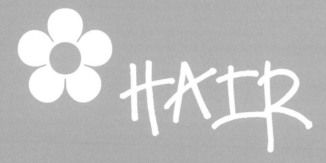

HAIR

Try going natural to achieve and mantain a healthy head of beautiful hair. These easy, all-natural recipes will help you clean, condition, brighten, lighten, or even darken your hair to the most flattering style for you .

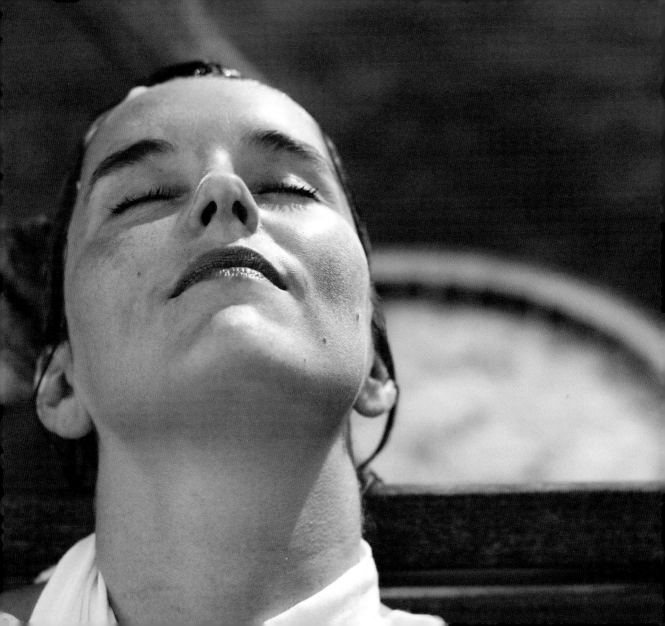

SHAMPOO

Commercial shampoos have made us accustomed to luscious sweet-scented lather. But lather has little to do with cleanliness. Soap herbs do not produce a foamy lather, just a light sudsy one.

HERBAL SOAPS

Soapwort

A pretty plant with pink flowers, smooth green stems and pointed leaves. It grows wild in temperate parts of the world and cultivated varieties can be found if you ask around. It likes rich, moist soil and some shade and is a very good plant to have in the garden both for its appearance and its use. The whole plant contains saponin—when the root, leaves and stems are boiled in water they give off a light soapy lather. If you don't grow your own herb, dried soapwort is obtainable at herbalists.

Yucca (The dried root is used.)

Soapbark (The dried bark is used.)

All you have to do is to pour hot water over a small amount of chopped herb and beat the water until suds form. Used alone the water makes a good, clean shampoo that leaves little residue on the hair. Mixed with an infusion of herbs it makes an even better one.

Herbal Shampoo

1. Pour 1 pint (475mL) of boiling water over a handful dried soapwort and leave, covered, to cool.
2. Meanwhile, make a strong cupful infusion of the herb most suited to your needs and leave that to cool. After about half an hour strain the soapwort and add the water to the infusion.

This makes a shampoo which is gently soapy and which conditions the hair. If you wish to make sure all vestige of shampoo is removed, tip some cider vinegar into the final rinsing water.

If soapwort, yucca or soapbark is unobtainable, mix together equal quantities baby shampoo and a very strong "tea" made from the herb of your choice. If you plan to use all the shampoo at one go you can beat in an egg and a squeeze of fresh aloe gel to give more shine and body. Leave out the egg if you wish to store the shampoo.

Dry Shampoo

Mix together equal quantities orris root powder and powdered arrowroot or corn flour and fuller's earth, and sprinkle over the hair, systematically using a comb to make sure all the hair is covered. Leave for about 15 minutes for the powder to absorb grease and dirt and then brush out (not with a nylon brush) until the hair looks clean and shiny.

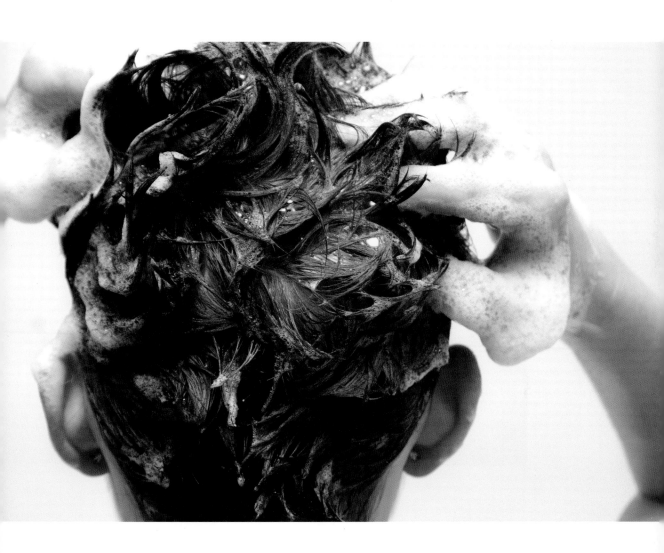

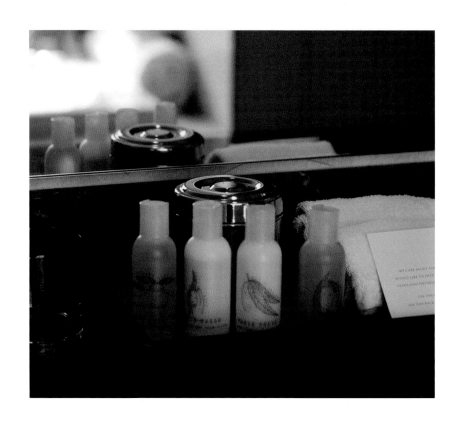

✿ NATURAL BODY CARE ✿

CONDITIONER

Hair Conditioner

Herbs can be steeped in oil and used as conditioners just as one steeps them in oil and uses them in cooking.

Put a quantity of bruised herbs suitable for your hair in a glass jar and cover them with oil—sunflower, safflower, peanut, or soya—olive oil if you are a brunette. Cover with muslin or other open cloth that will let air through and put the jar somewhere warm, out of direct heat and where the temperature does not drop dramatically. Leave for at least a fortnight, shaking the jar each day. Strain, pressing the herbs with a spoon to get all the oil out of them. Bottle and add a nice label.

Oils for conditioning can be slightly warmed, rubbed through the hair, and massaged into the scalp.

When the oil has been applied, put on a plastic bath cap, wrap head in a warm towel and relax in a warm place for half an hour or so. Change towel for another warm one if it cools too quickly.

Light Conditioner

1 tablespoon each of lanolin, glycerin and almond oil
3 drops rosemary oil
1 egg (beaten)

1. Warm and combine all ingredients except the egg. Mix thoroughly.
2. Beat in the beaten egg.
3. Using the fingers, stroke the conditioner through the hair and massage into the scalp. Put on a bath cap and sit and enjoy a cup of tea then rinse the hair thoroughly with warm water.

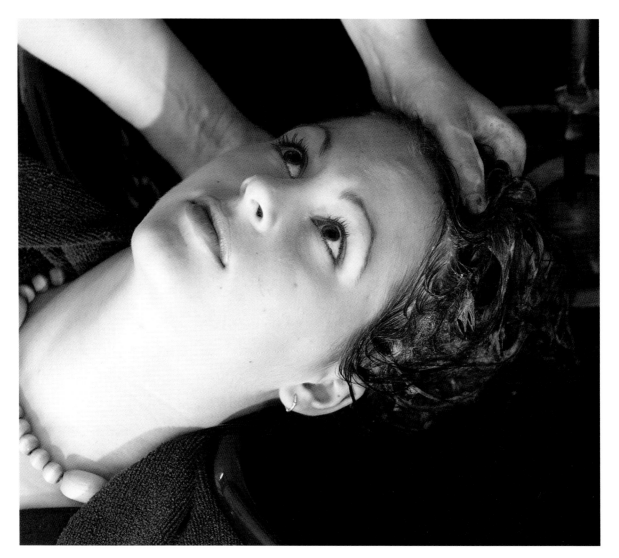

✿ NATURAL BODY CARE ✿

RINSES AND DYES

Rinse for Fair Hair

Make a strong tea from a mixture of dried chamomile, marigold, and lemon verbena flowers. When cool, rinse through the hair several times.

Rinse for Dark Hair

Make a strong tea from a mixture of sage and rosemary leaves. When cool, rinse through the hair several times. Or save the remains of a pot of Indian tea and use that as a rinse.

For red hair, a tea made from marigold petals is a good rinse.

Dyeing Hair

Henna is one of the oldest natural cosmetic dyes. The dye is produced by mixing water with crushed henna leaves. Sometimes lemon juice, indigo leaves, herbs, essential oils, vinegar, and oil are added to create different dyes.

Henna has proved over the years that it does not injure the hair. The color it can produce when used in inexperienced hands, however, has been known to create a great deal of dismay. Henna is for the fun-loving prepared to take a chance.

If you buy henna powder for home use, ask for instructions as to how to use it and stick to them. The color you create will last for up to three months.

Henna is actually quite good for the hair; it adds fullness and luster and does not attack the natural pigment. If you really want to "go henna" begin by going to a professional and learn exactly how to get it right.

Sadly, if you do use it and hate the result you will have to wait until the hennaed hair has grown out before you can safely re-dye it or have a permanent wave.

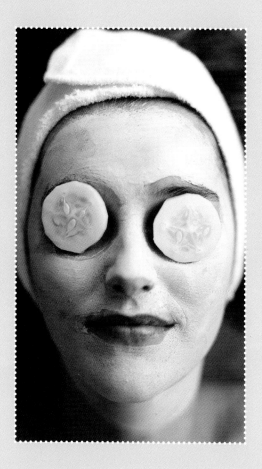
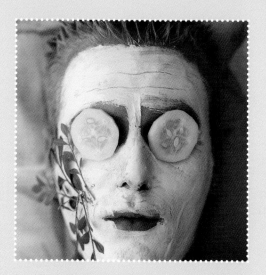
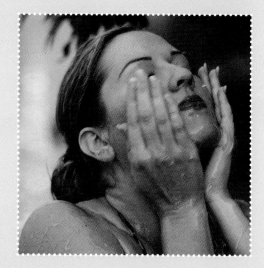

EYES

The skin around the eyes is much thinner than the skin on the rest of your face and requires more attention and care to ward off the signs of aging. For all eye care, eight hours sleep is essential as well 8–10 full glasses of water every day.

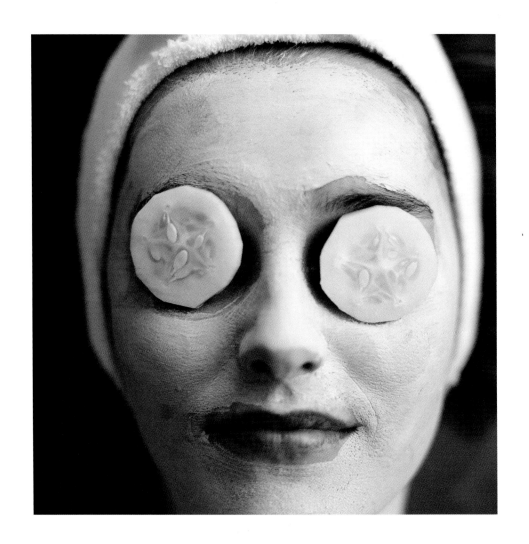

DARK CIRCLES

Lack of sleep, fatigue, or simply aging can cause dark circles under the eyes. Follow the steps below for a full eye treatment.

Cucumber Eye Pads

2 slices raw cucumber, ¼ inch thick

eye cream

Cover each closed eyelid with a slice of the cucumber. Leave for 15–20 minutes. Rinse with warm water. Gently pat eye cream (never drag the skin) along the bone directly under the eye avoiding contact with eye.

Face Mask

vitamin E capsule

½ teaspoon honey

1 beaten egg white

Mix honey and egg white. Rub powdered vitamin E capsule along the bone directly under the eye. Wipe off with honey and egg white mix.

Chamomile Eye Pads

cold chamomile tea

2 cotton-wool pads

face mask

Soak pads in chamomile tea. While relaxing with your face mask on, place pads on your eyes. After removing mask, rinse eyes with warm water.

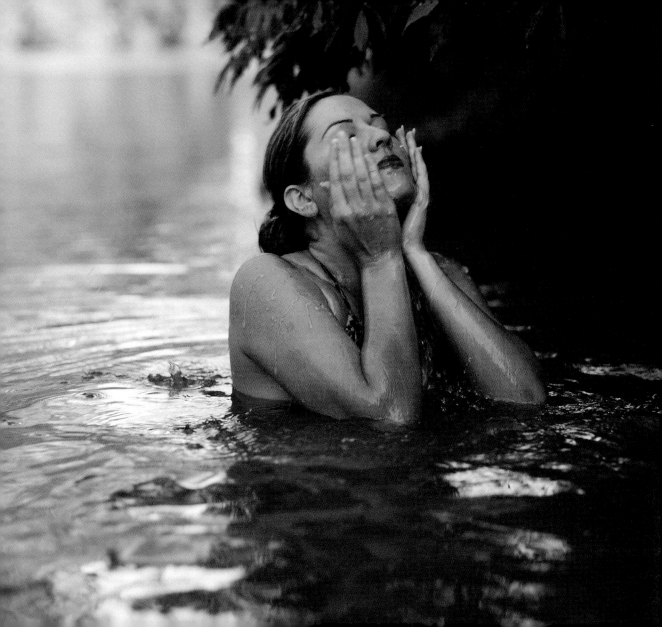

PUFFINESS

Puffiness is caused by a build-up of toxins and excess fluids. This is a relatively simple process to soothe the eyes and decrease the swelling.

Use your middle finger to stimulate the lymphatic system by pressing gently on the skin around the eyes. Start on the brow bone and work your way along the outside of the eye and along the orbital bone (the bone directly under the eye). You can also store a jar of eye cream in the fridge and gently pat it onto the skin around your eyes while stimulating the lymphatic system. This will help to cool and soothe while decreasing the puffiness.

SORE EYES

This eye bath will help to soothe sore eyes caused by exposure to the elements. When you are purchasing rose water, be sure to buy only the 100 percent pure form, as there are no added preservatives.

1–2 tablespoons rose water
⅔ cup (150mL) distilled water

Mix the rose water with the distilled water. Gently bathe the eyes with the mixture and then softly pat dry.

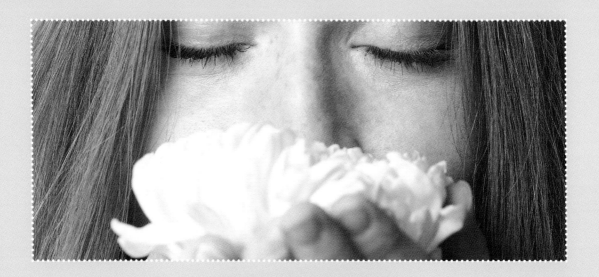
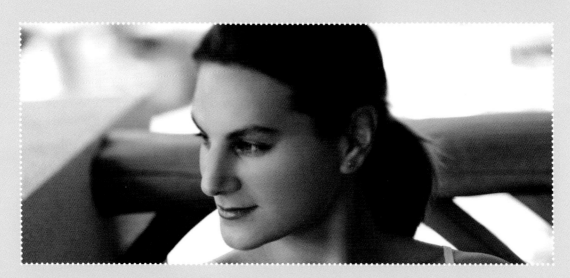

MIND

While stress is arguably the number one health issue in modern life, learning to relax and calm our minds should be one of our highest priorities. Follow these simple techniques to add a little relief into your hectic schedule.

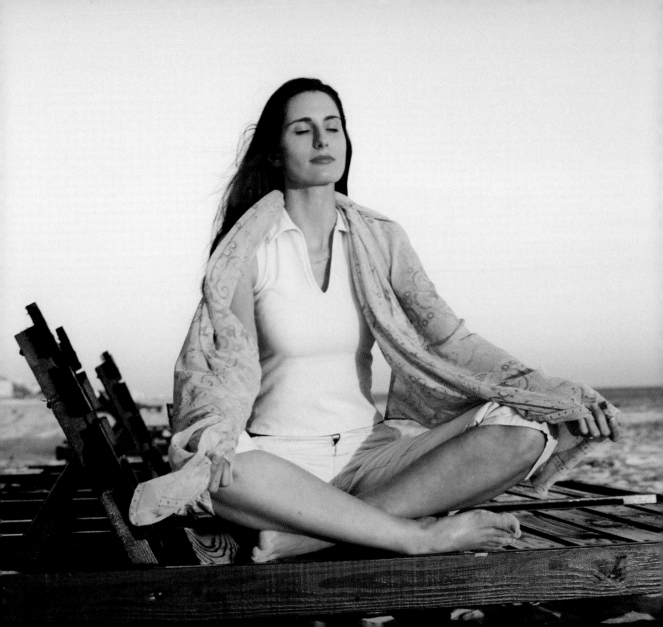

MEDITATION

Meditation is the best thing you can do for your body. It is a wonderful way to counter stress, calm your mind, and bring serenity and clarity. The practice has many health benefits as well. It can help lower cholesterol, ease chronic pain, end insomnia, boost the immune system, counter anxiety, and improve circulation. Since meditation requires unbroken attention on one thing, find the best position that helps you stay focused and relaxed.

Basic Breathing Meditiation

Practice this technique daily for a week for 10 minutes. Work your way up to 15 and then 20 minutes five to seven days a week.

1. Sit comfortably, legs crossed, back straight, and arms resting on your knees about 45 degrees from your torso.
2. Breathe through your nose. Feel and observe where each breath is moving through your body.
3. Notice the changes of the breath as you give it your awareness. Notice how your awareness changes and you notice the breath.
4. Focus on the breath. If your attention drifts, bring it softly back to focusing on the breath.
5. As you become accustomed to this technique, bring the breath into other areas of the body (such as the small of your back) that feel dull. Allow it to follow your consciousness, don't force it, to those dull areas.
6. When your session is complete, gently stretch out your legs and arms.

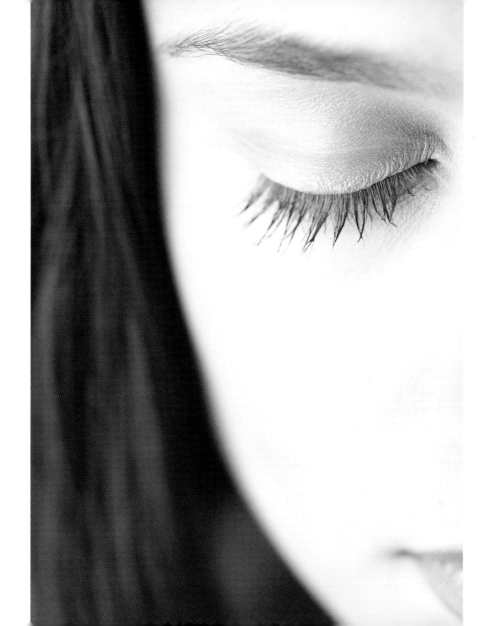

Listening Meditation

This type of meditation allows you to focus outward rather than inward. Try this technique for 5 minutes to begin, then add a minute or two until you can reach a full 20 minutes.

1. Sit comfortably with your eyes closed and focus on each breath for a few minutes.
2. Slowly bring your awareness to the sounds around you. The goal is to simply "hear" the sounds; the quiet, dominant, and even the silences without focusing on one or the other. If you find yourself identifying sounds, you need to gently re-direct your focus back to the sounds.
3. To end the session, slowly open your eyes and stand.

cold chamomile tea
2 cotton-wool pads
face mask

Soak pads in chamomile tea. While relaxing with your face mask on, place pads on your eyes. After removing mask, rinse eyes with warm water.

RELAXATION

Relaxation is a fantastic way to slow down and reduce the effects of daily stress. True relaxation can be achieved through structured, simple things. There are a variety of ways to attain deep relaxation from simple yoga techniques to a warm, scented bath. A few of the benefits include: relief of lower back pain, lower blood pressure, and decreased fatigue.

Basic Relaxation Pose

For this pose you will need:
5 folded blankets
4 small pillows
cotton face cloth

1. Lie down on your back on a comfortable surface. Support your lower legs and backs of your knees with the towels, keeping your shins parallel to the floor. Place a towel under each wrist and rest your elbows on the floor. With the rest of the pillows, support your shoulders, neck and head. Cover your eyes with the face cloth.
2. Release the tension in your body by imagining you are sinking into the floor. Take slow, deep breaths and relax. Focus on your breathing to the exclusion of all else. Continue for 5–10 minutes.
3. To finish, bend one knee, roll to your side, and sit up.

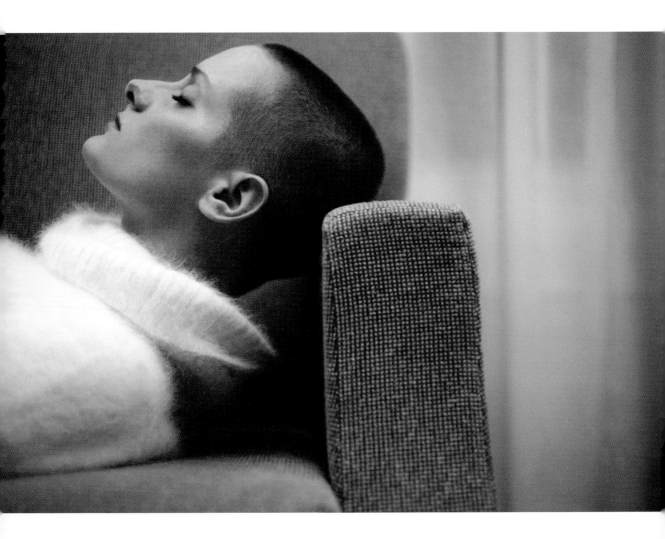

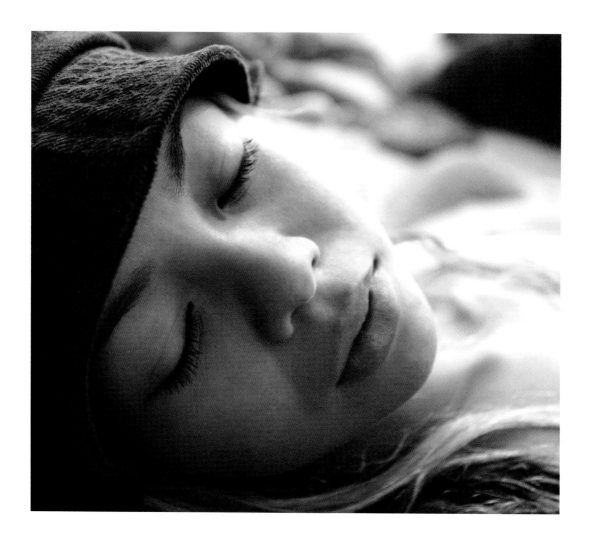

✿ NATURAL BODY CARE ✿

Deepest Relaxation Pose

For this pose you will need:
2 small pillows
1 large pillow
cotton face cloth

1. Lie down on your back on a comfortable surface. Support your neck and shoulders with a small pillow. Support your knees with the large pillow and your ankles with the smaller one. Cover your eyes with the face cloth.

2. Begin by slowly inhaling and exhaling. After a few minutes, return to a more natural rhythm of breathing. Focus on relaxing every bone, muscle, and organ in your body. Focus inward, concentrating on each part of your body as you unwind.

3. To finish the pose, bend your knees and roll gently to your side. Slowly sit up.

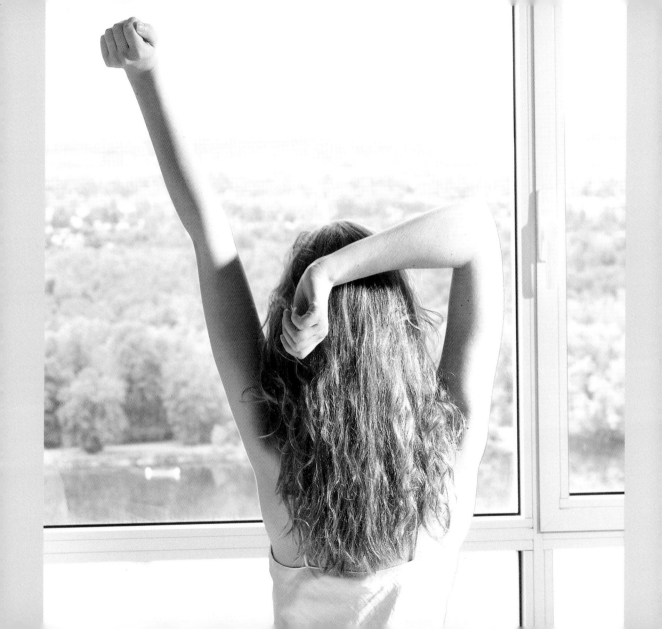

VITALITY

We all need a little more vitality physically, mentally, and emotionally. Sometimes all it takes is allowing ourselves the time to energize inside and out. Building vitality will help to improve your emotional health as well as your odds against chronic illness, immunity to infection, balance, strength and flexibility, and mental sharpness.

When You Arise

• Drink in the sun. Welcome the new day by throwing back the curtains. Sunlight inhibits the release of melatonin (the sleepy hormone), giving your energy levels and mood a pick-me-up.

• Yawn. The brain receives more oxygen by yawning, increasing mental clarity.

• Take a moment to breathe. Inhale and exhale slowly for a few minutes. This will clear your head and help you focus while relieving stress.

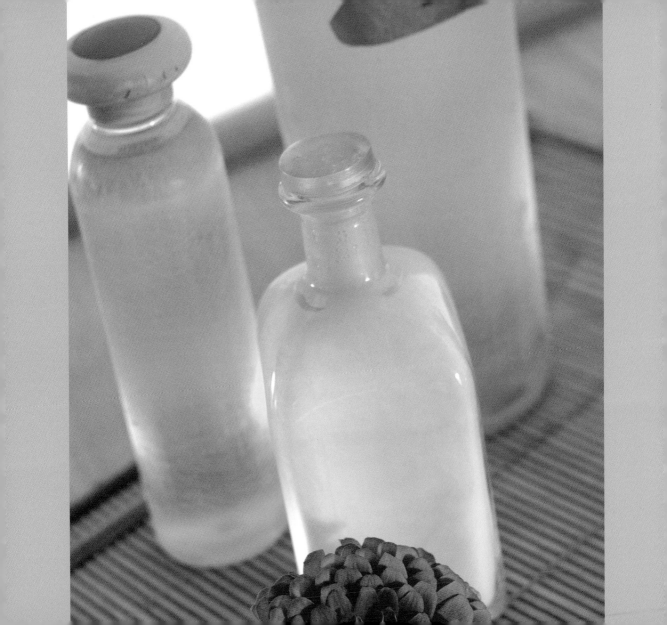

AROMATHERAPY

Aromatherapy is therapeutic for your mind and body. In the home, essential oils can be used in a variety of ways for their fragrance and for their medicinal qualities. Since they are easily absorbed through the skin, directly into the blood stream, they are considered very powerful and should only be used in diluted form; in a bath, sprinkled in a shower tray, diluted in almond oil for massage, or in an aromatic diffuser. Using essential oils will awaken your senses and restore your energy.

Energizing Essential Oils

Lemon
Lifts the spirits and boosts the immune system

Bergamot
Relieves fatigue, depression, and melancholy

Ginger
Revives vital energy

Juniper
Can be used to eliminate toxins from the body

Rosemary
Raises energy levels

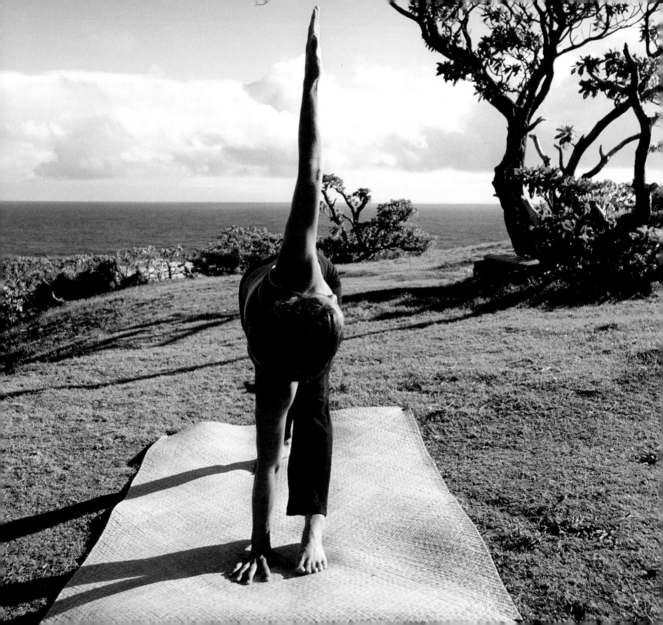

YOGA

Imagine that in just a few minutes a day you could relieve stress, relax your body, and clear your mind. Yoga is practiced in many forms from modern yoga, which is an energetic workout, to traditional yoga, which is done with simple postures. Yoga is designed to achieve a deep relaxation and concentration.

Cobra Pose

This technique works wonders for relieving tension in the lower back while improving your posture.

1. Lie on a comfortable surface on your stomach. Point your kneecaps at the floor and place your feet 1 foot apart.
2. Slowly lower your forehead to the floor and extend your arms out to your sides with palms facing inward.
3. Take a deep breath. As you exhale, lower your shoulder blades down toward your waist. Take another deep breath; exhale and raise your arms up and back toward your feet, lifting into an arch. Look slightly down keeping your legs on the floor.
4. Hold for 3–5 breaths. Slowly lower your arms and shoulders, resting your forehead on the floor. Repeat twice.

Half Forward Fold

This pose will stretch your hamstrings, calf muscles, and lower back while also working your quadriceps. Try using this technique before or after walking or running.

1. Stand facing a wall 6 feet away. Your feet should be parallel and hip-width apart. Extend your arms out in front of you and rest your palms on the wall just above waist level.
2. Inhale, and as you exhale, walk your feet back, bending at the hips. Your torso should be parallel to the ground, your back flat.
3. Pushing through your feet, tighten your quadriceps and pull your thighs back. You should feel the stretch through your hamstrings and lower back. Hold for 5–7 breaths.
4. To end the pose, walk back toward the wall with your knees bent slightly and stand up.

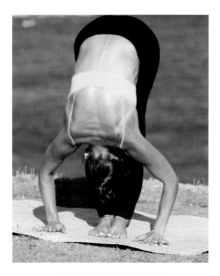

❀ NATURAL BODY CARE ❀

Extended Triangle Pose

This pose will strengthen the legs, stretch the groins, hamstrings, hips, and open the chest and shoulders.

1. Stand erect; place the feet apart slightly more than shoulder width. Keep the feet in line, pointing forward. Balance the weight of the body evenly between the two feet. Keep the head straight. Pivot on your heel, rotating right foot out 90 degrees. The heel of the right foot lines up with the arch of the left foot. Inhale deeply. Open the chest; stretch the arms wide on the sides in line with the shoulders and parallel to the ground. Open palms and stretch the fingers. Breathe.

2. While exhaling and relaxing the whole body, lean to your right side by rotating the pelvis and turning the trunk slightly up towards the ceiling, and bringing the right hand fingers down touching the floor near the outer side of the foot. If possible, the right palm should rest completely on the floor.

3. Now stretch the left arm up, bringing it in line with the right arm, and lengthening the spine. Look at the palm of the outstretched left hand with the corner of the eye. Keep the arms, shoulders, hips, and back of the legs aligned in a vertical plane. Take some deep inhales and exhales while the mind observes the movements of the breath.

4. Face down, with deep inhaling and relaxing, slowly come-up by reversing the steps (3, 2, and 1). Repeat the steps on the left side. Do not bend the knees or elbows when leaning down or getting up.

Silverleaf Press Books are available exclusively

through Independent Publishers Group.

For details write or telephone

Independent Publishers Group, 814 North Franklin St.

Chicago, IL 60610, (312) 337-0747

Silverleaf Press

8160 South Highland Drive

Sandy, Utah 84093

ISBN: 978-1-933317-74-8

MEDAL
OF HONOR

JOHN PERRITANO

red rhino
bOOks®
NONFICTION

Photo credits: page 1: Chuck Franklin / Alamy Stock Photo; page 2/3: PJF Military Collection / Alamy Stock Photo; page 9: Everett Historical / Shutterstock.com; page 10: Oriole Gin / Shutterstock.com; page 12: SueC / Shutterstock.com; page 13: Joseph Sohm / Shutterstock.com; page 16/17: Everett Historical / Shutterstock.com; page 20: James Kirkikis / Shutterstock.com; page 23: Stocktrek Images, Inc. / Alamy Stock Photo; page 29: neftali / Shutterstock.com; page 36: LandFox / Shutterstock.com; page 39: 615 collection / Alamy Stock Photo; page 41: PJF Military Collection / Alamy Stock Photo; page 47: 615 collection / Alamy Stock Photo; All other source images from Shutterstock.com

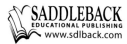

SADDLEBACK
EDUCATIONAL PUBLISHING
www.sdlback.com

ISBN-13: 978-1-68021-054-5
ISBN-10: 1-68021-054-8
eBook: 978-1-63078-373-0

Printed in Malaysia

22 21 20 19 18   1 2 3 4 5

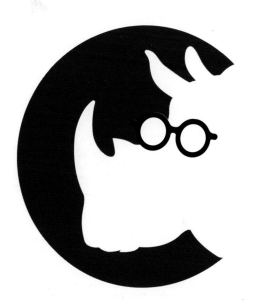

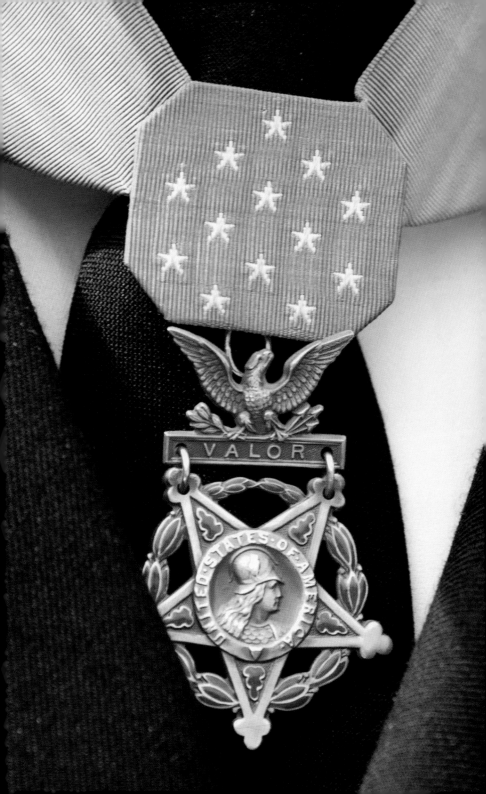

TABLE OF CONTENTS

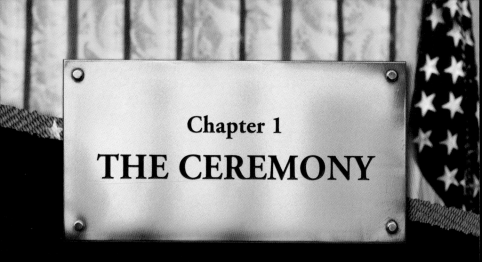

Chapter 1
THE CEREMONY

It was June 2, 2015.

There was an event.

It was at the White House.

President Obama spoke.

He held a case.

A medal was inside.

It was the *Medal of Honor*.

This is a US military honor.

It is the top one.

Obama talked about two men.

Both were *soldiers*.

They fought in World War I.

William Shemin was one.

Henry Johnson was the other.

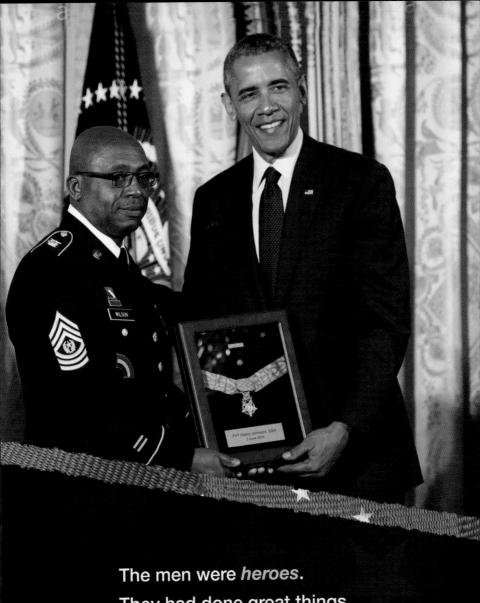

The men were *heroes*.

They had done great things.

Shemin saved many lives.

Johnson did too.

Both had been *wounded*.

The men deserved the Medal of Honor.

They got other awards.

France gave Johnson one.

It was France's top award for *valor*.

Johnson was the first American to get it.

But neither got the Medal of Honor.

Why not?

Shemin was Jewish.

Johnson was African American.

It was almost a century later.

Many thought this day would never come.

It finally did.

"We remember our heroes," Obama said.

"It's never too late to say thank you."

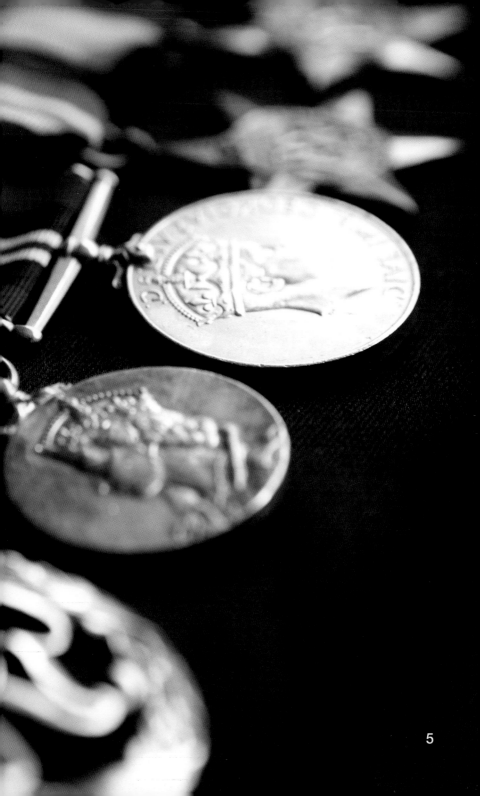

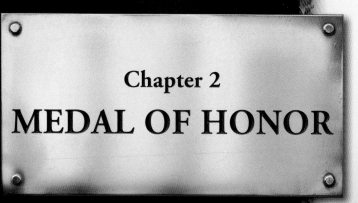

Chapter 2
MEDAL OF HONOR

Soldiers are heroes.
They answer a call.
It is to serve the country.

Some go above and beyond.
Many *honor* them.
Medals are one way.
The US gives the Medal of Honor.

The award began in 1861.
It was for valor.
Not every soldier gets this.
Only the bravest do.

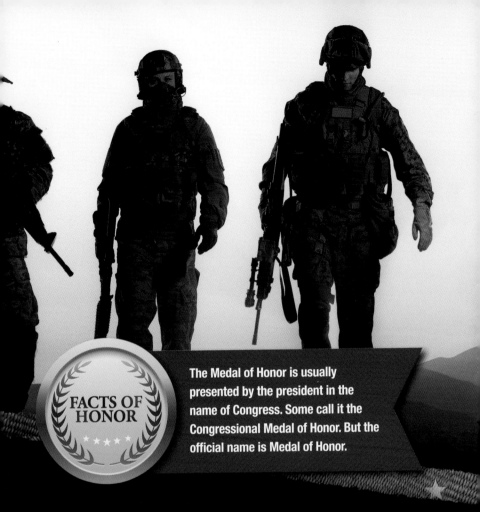

FACTS OF HONOR

The Medal of Honor is usually presented by the president in the name of Congress. Some call it the Congressional Medal of Honor. But the official name is Medal of Honor.

Sometimes the person has died.

They can still get one.

Family gets the medal.

The first one was given in 1863.

More than 3,500 have one.

Here are some of their stories.

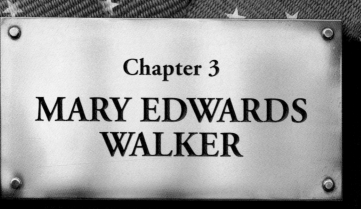

Chapter 3

MARY EDWARDS WALKER

It was 1861.

The Civil War had begun.

Mary Edwards Walker wanted to help.

She helped the *Union*.

Walker was a doctor.

But she could not work as one.

The Army had a rule.

Women could not be doctors.

She worked as a nurse.

Walker worked in a hospital.

She helped troops.

Some were sick.

Others had been hurt.

Later she went to the field.

There were tent hospitals.

She worked there.

Then the Army made a change.

They let her be a surgeon.

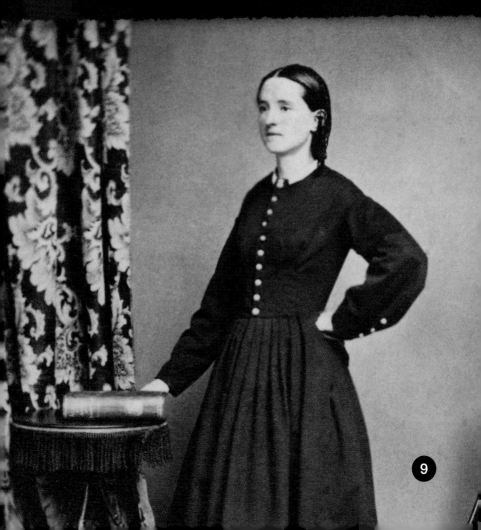

It was April 1864.
Walker crossed enemy lines.
Troops were hurt.
She was trying to help.
But some thought she was a spy.
She was taken prisoner.
The enemy held her.
They kept her for five months.
Then they let her go.

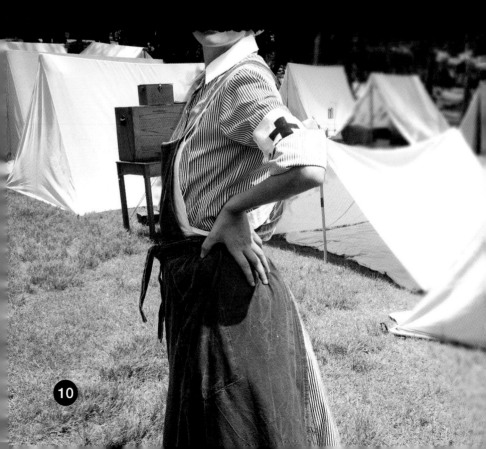

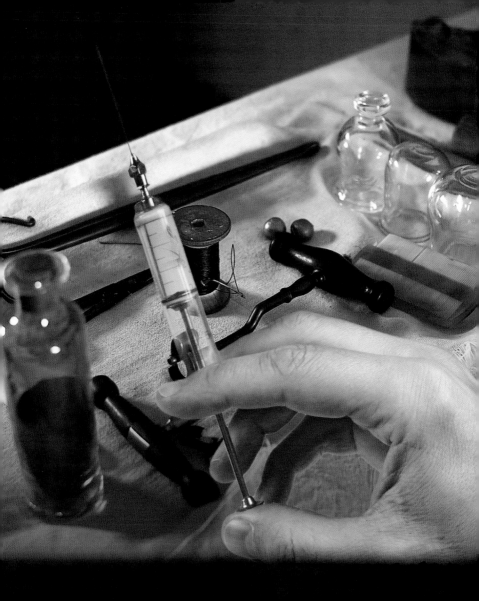

She went to work in a hospital.

It was for female prisoners.

Walker ran the hospital.

She also did surgery.

Finally the war ended.

Walker got the Medal of Honor.

She became famous.

Walker used her fame for change.

Back then, women could not vote.

Walker thought it was wrong.

She fought for their *rights*.

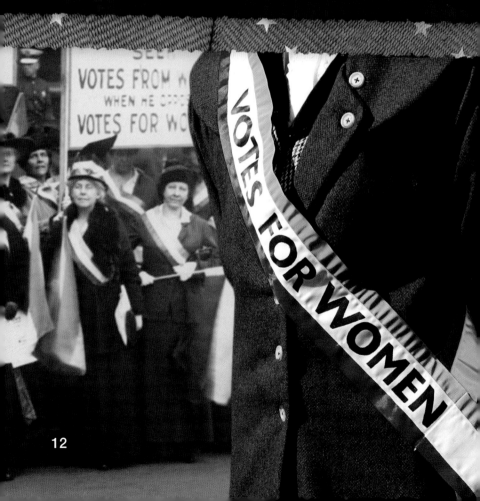

It was 1917.

The Army changed the rules.

Only soldiers could get the award.

Her name was taken off the list.

But she kept her medal.

Walker wore it until she died.

It was 1977.

President Carter restored her award.

Walker was put back on the list.

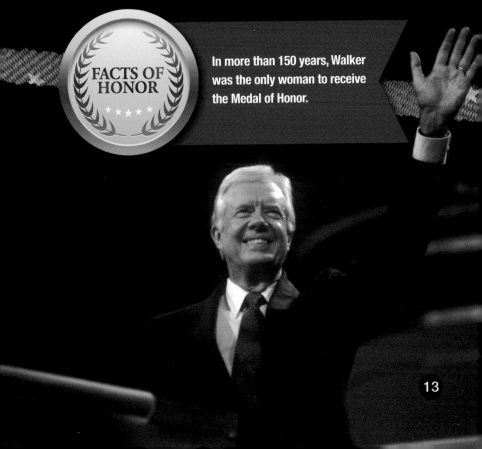

FACTS OF HONOR

In more than 150 years, Walker was the only woman to receive the Medal of Honor.

Chapter 4

WILLIAM CARNEY JR.

William Carney Jr. was a slave.

His parents were slaves too.

Carney's dad got away.

He used the *Underground Railroad*.

Then he got a job.

He saved his pay.

Finally there was enough money.

He paid to free his family.

His wife and son joined him.

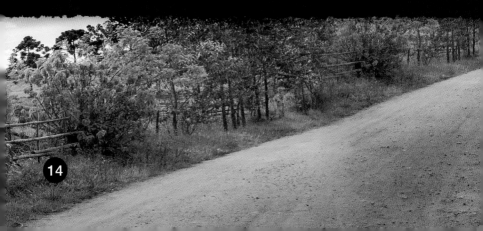

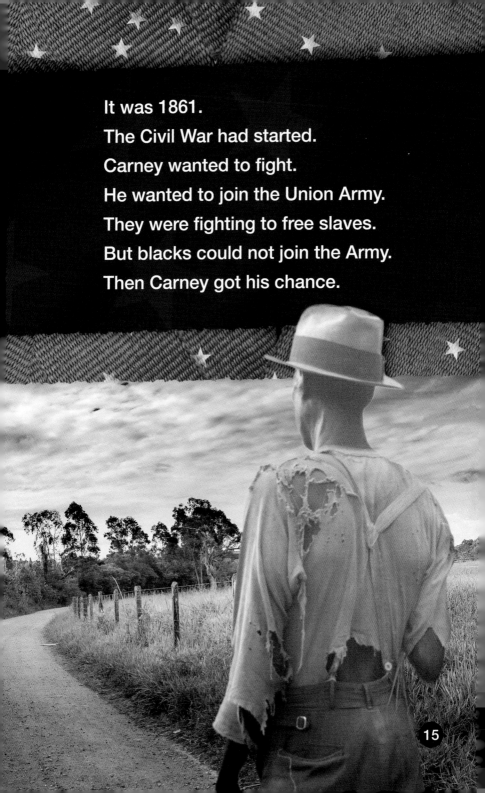

It was 1861.

The Civil War had started.

Carney wanted to fight.

He wanted to join the Union Army.

They were fighting to free slaves.

But blacks could not join the Army.

Then Carney got his chance.

15

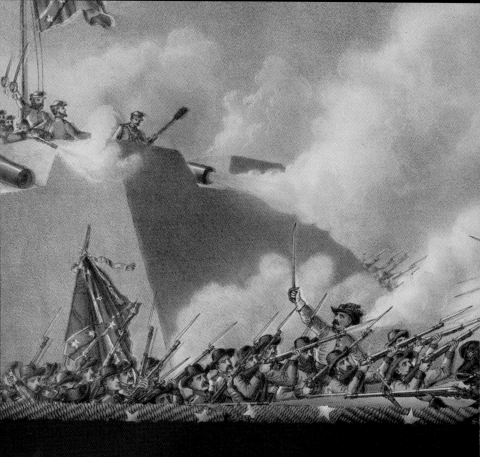

It was 1863.
There was a black unit.
It was called the 54th.
Carney joined.

The time came to fight.
The 54th was ready.
They were to storm Fort Wagner.
It was near Charleston, South Carolina.

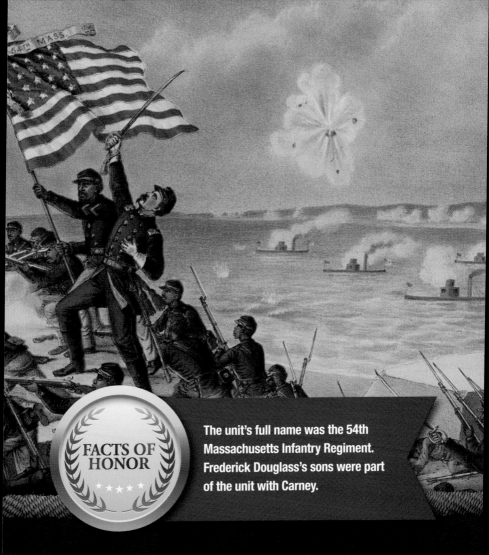

FACTS OF HONOR

The unit's full name was the 54th Massachusetts Infantry Regiment. Frederick Douglass's sons were part of the unit with Carney.

The battle started.

Cannons fired.

Shells exploded.

The 54th came from the coast.

They marched in.

Sand dunes were used for cover.

They neared the fort.
Troops waited for dark.
That is when they would attack.

Exploding shells lit up the sky.
The order came.
Troops charged.
One carried the American flag.
A bullet cut him down.
Carney saw it happen.
He did not want the flag to fall.

Carney dropped his gun.
He grabbed the flag.
It waved high.
He stood alone on the fort's wall.

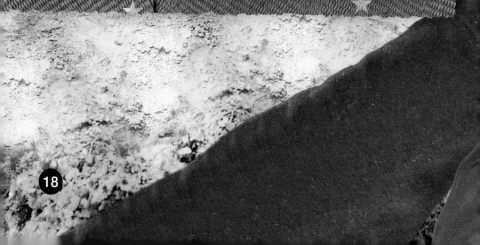

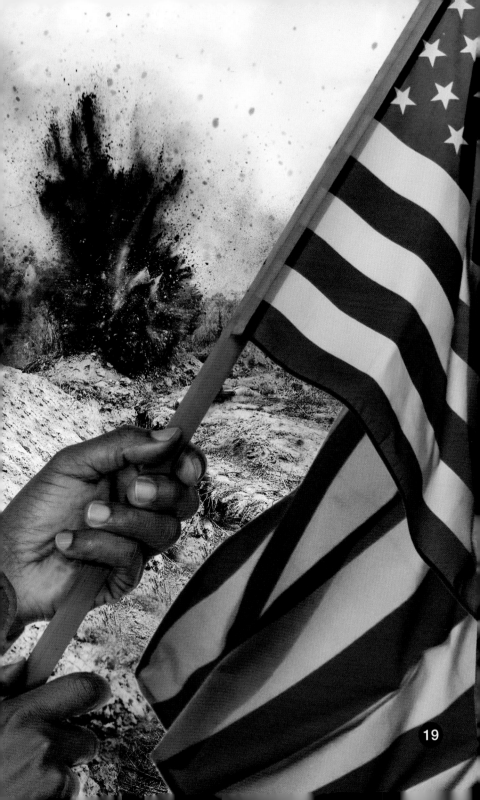

Bullets flew.

Carney was hurt.

Bullets hit him all over.

But he kept the flag up.

This gave the 54th hope.

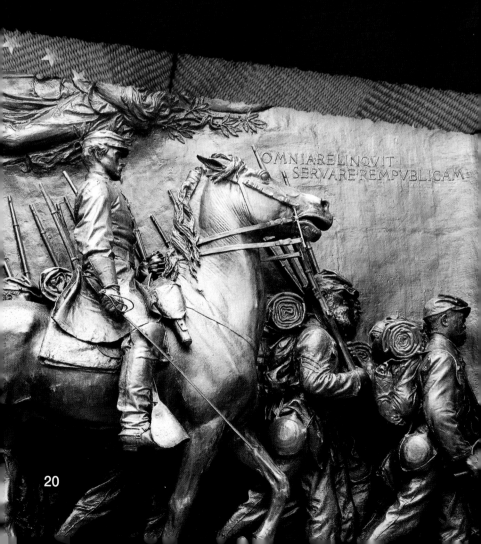

The battle was a mess.

Many of the 54th died.

But Carney did not.

He was hurt.

But he never let go of the flag.

He brought it back to his unit.

"The old flag never touched the ground."

Some said black troops could not fight.

The 54th proved them wrong.

Carney was a hero.

The Medal of Honor was his prize.

He was the first African American to get one.

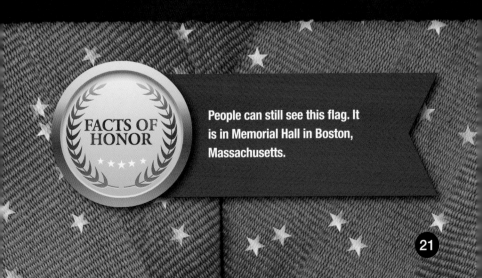

FACTS OF HONOR

People can still see this flag. It is in Memorial Hall in Boston, Massachusetts.

Chapter 5

JOHN BASILONE

It was the summer of 1942.

The US was at war.

This was World War II.

Marines were in the Pacific.

They went to islands.

Their goal was to secure them.

They kept the enemy away.

Guadalcanal was a tiny island.

It had an *airstrip*.

The Japanese were there.

Their planes used it.

The planes fought the US.

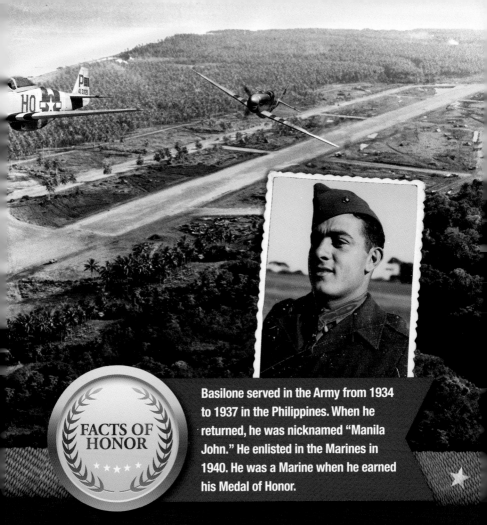

It was August 7, 1942.

The Marines invaded.

They stormed the beach.

The enemy went into the mountains.

They hid and waited.

The battle would be long.

It would last until February 1943.

It was October 24.

John Basilone led two units.

They were machine *gunners*.

There were 16 of them.

They had four machine guns.

Darkness fell.

The enemy attacked.

The gunners fought back hard.

Fighting was fierce.

Many Japanese were killed.

So were Marines.

Bodies piled up.

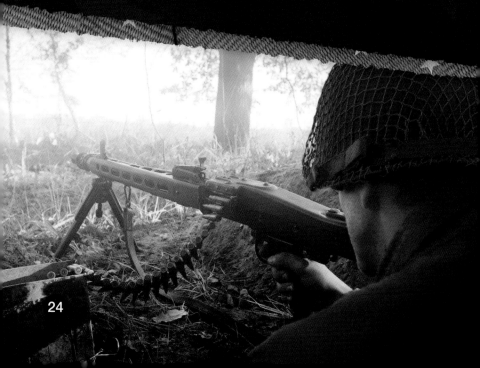

Two gunners were left.

Only one gun worked.

Basilone gave them an order.

Keep the gun loaded.

Do not stop firing.

He repaired another gun.

The three men held the line.

Supply lines were cut off.

Shells ran low.

The gunners needed more.

Basilone ran through heavy fire.

He came back with more shells.

Fighting did not stop.

Shells ran low again.

Basilone went for more.

He ran through heavy fire again.

The fight went on all night.
Then the sun came up.
Almost 3,000 Japanese were dead.
The rest retreated.
They left the island.

Basilone was a hero.
He received the Medal of Honor.

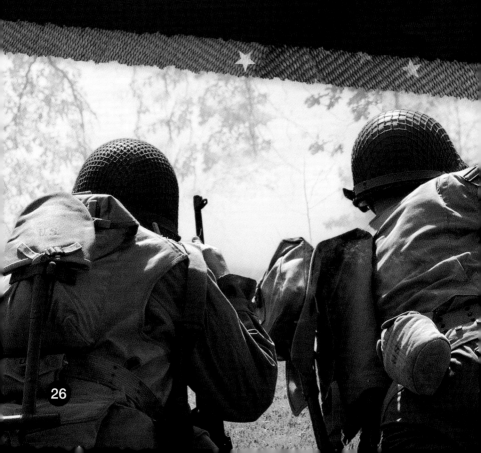

Basilone went back home.

He made speeches.

The medal was on his chest.

He asked people to support the war.

But he wanted to fight.

He got his chance.

His unit was sent back to the Pacific.

He was killed in Iwo Jima.

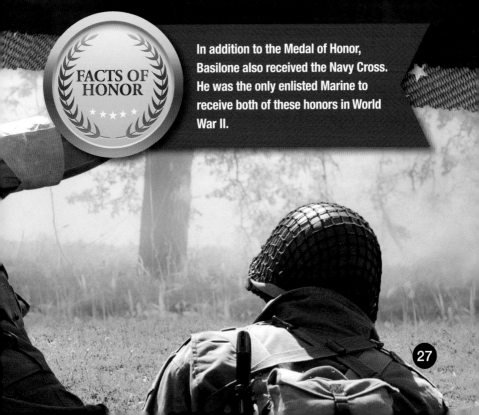

FACTS OF HONOR

In addition to the Medal of Honor, Basilone also received the Navy Cross. He was the only enlisted Marine to receive both of these honors in World War II.

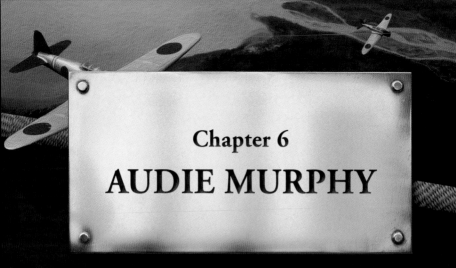

Chapter 6
AUDIE MURPHY

It was 1942.

World War II was in full swing.

Pearl Harbor had been hit.

Audie Murphy was mad.

He wanted to fight.

But he was only 17.

He was too young.

The Army would not take him.

He faked his records.

His age was changed.

The Army let him in.

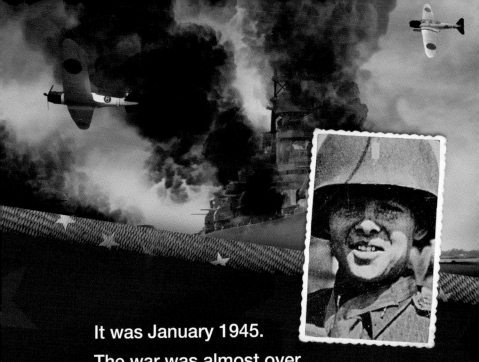

It was January 1945.

The war was almost over.

Murphy was in France.

He was near the German border.

The Germans held a town.

It was called Holtzwihr.

Murphy's company had 120 men.

They moved to the town.

The Germans fought back.

They killed 102 of the men.

Murphy was the only officer alive.

He was wounded.

But he took charge.

29

The German attack continued.
The enemy had six *tanks*.
They had 250 troops.
Murphy knew things were bad.
He told his men to fall back.
They went to safer ground.

Murphy stayed.
He faced the enemy alone.
A tank burned nearby.
Murphy climbed aboard.
He aimed its machine guns.
The guns blasted.

Murphy killed many.
The rest surrounded him.
But he would not give up.
He kept firing.
Then the shells ran out.

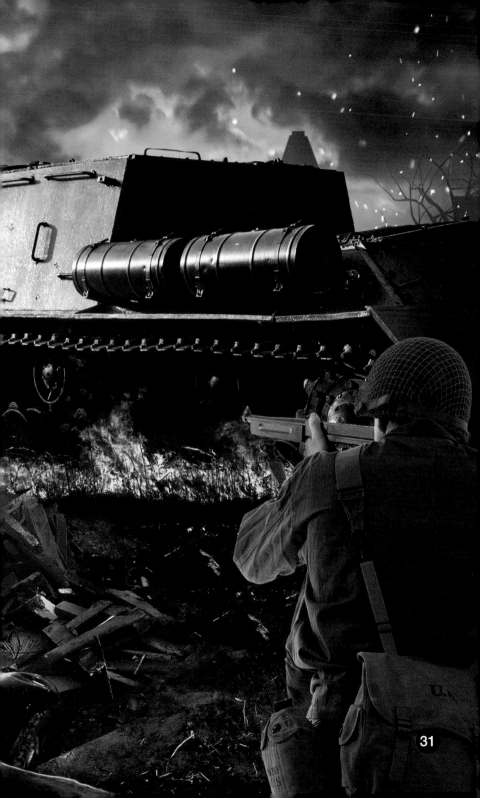

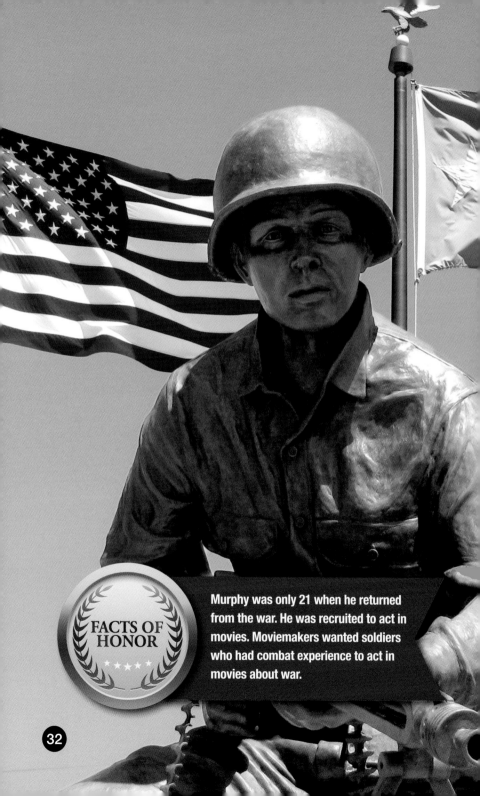

FACTS OF HONOR

Murphy was only 21 when he returned from the war. He was recruited to act in movies. Moviemakers wanted soldiers who had combat experience to act in movies about war.

Murphy retreated.

He joined his men.

His body was wounded.

But he ignored that.

He took charge again.

Murphy gave an order.

He told his men to attack.

They fought back the Germans.

Finally the Germans left.

Murphy saved many lives that day.

He got 33 awards.

No other World War II soldier had more.

The Medal of Honor was the top one.

Murphy came home.

His story made him famous.

He became a movie star.

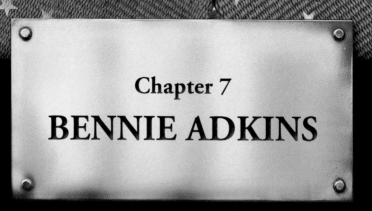

Chapter 7
BENNIE ADKINS

Vietnam was at war.

The North was fighting the South.

The US was an ally of the South.

It was March 9, 1966.

The North attacked a camp.

No one knew it yet.

But the battle would last 38 hours.

Bennie Adkins had a *mortar*.

He fired at the enemy.

The enemy fired back at him.

He was hurt.

Troops were hurt too.

Adkins ran to them.

He dragged them to safety.

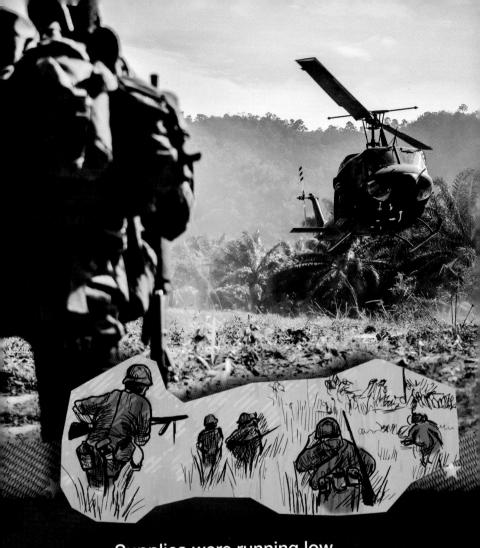

Supplies were running low.

A *chopper* had dropped some.

They landed in a field.

It was full of mines.

Adkins went to get them.

It meant leaving the camp.

He brought the supplies back.

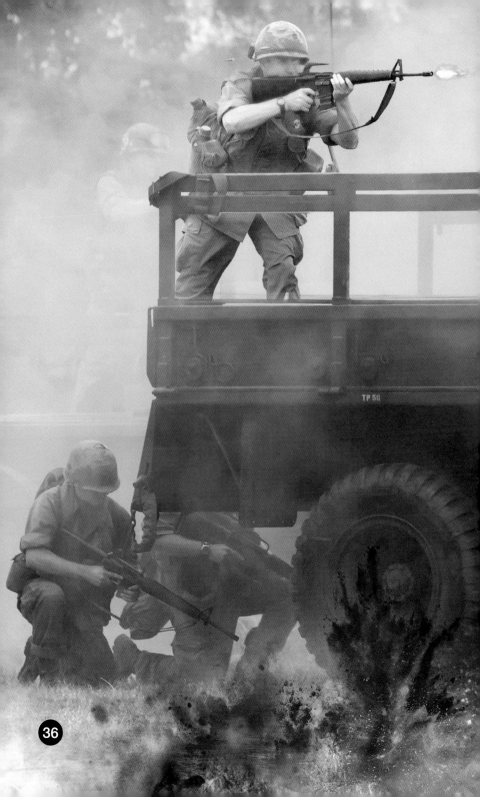

Fighting went on.

The next day was worse.

A big attack came from the North.

Many wounded needed help.

Adkins drew enemy fire.

He wanted them to target him.

There was a reason.

Help could get to the wounded.

The enemy broke through.

They stormed the camp.

There were waves of them.

Adkins kept firing.

He fired until shells were gone.

A *bunker* was nearby.

Adkins led troops there.

They dug their way out.

Troops ran into the jungle.

Choppers were there.

They could rescue them.

But time ran out.

The choppers had to go.

Troops were stuck.

They kept moving.

The enemy chased them.

This went on for two days.

There was a tiger there too.

He stalked them all.

The enemy was worried.

They were scared of the tiger.

Finally they left.

They let the troops be.

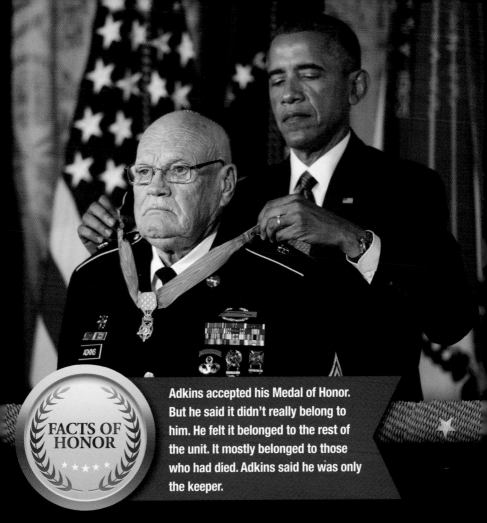

FACTS OF HONOR

Adkins accepted his Medal of Honor. But he said it didn't really belong to him. He felt it belonged to the rest of the unit. It mostly belonged to those who had died. Adkins said he was only the keeper.

Adkins got away.

Many others did too.

He was hurt 18 times.

But that did not stop him.

"You just don't quit," he said.

Adkins got the Medal of Honor.

Chapter 8

ROSS A. McGINNIS

It was 2003.

US troops were in Iraq.

Other countries were there too.

Ross McGinnis joined the Army.

That was the next year.

Soon he left for Iraq.

It was December 4, 2006.

McGinnis was on *patrol*.

He was on a truck.

His job was to watch behind it.

His gun was ready to fire.

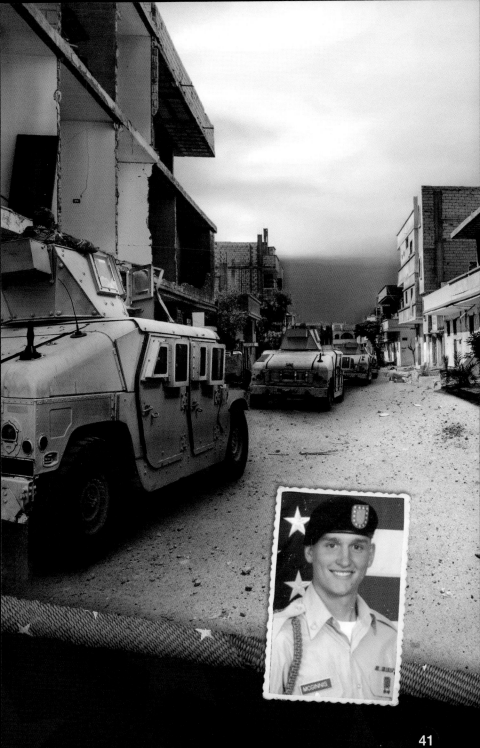

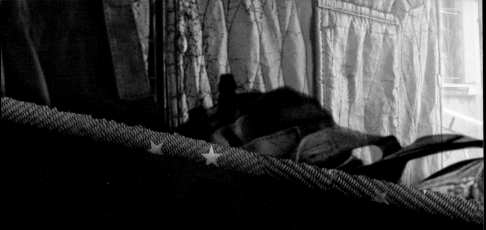

An enemy threw a *grenade*.

It fell into the truck.

McGinnis yelled a warning.

There was no time.

They were trapped.

The grenade was about to blow.

He jumped on it.

It cost him his life.

But the troops with him lived.

There were four of them.

He had saved their lives.

McGinnis was a hero.

He got the Medal of Honor.

His family accepted it.

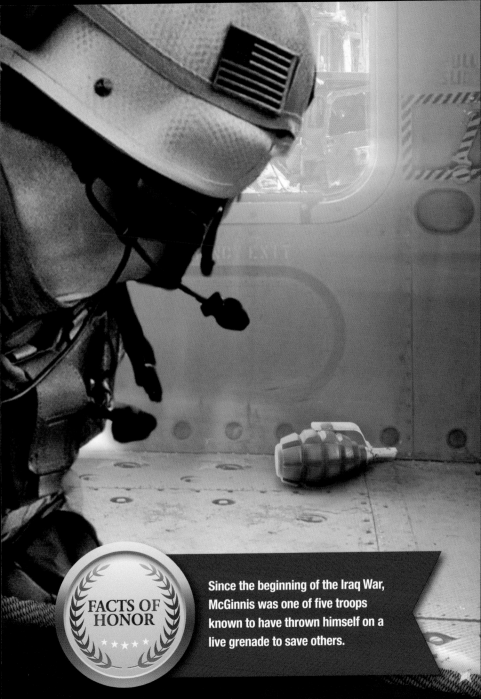

FACTS OF HONOR

Since the beginning of the Iraq War, McGinnis was one of five troops known to have thrown himself on a live grenade to save others.

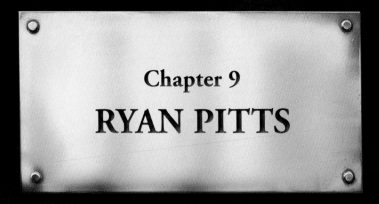

Chapter 9
RYAN PITTS

It was 2008.

Troops were in Afghanistan.

A US base was hit.

The enemy was armed.

They had machine guns.

Rockets fired grenades.

Ryan Pitts was on *duty*.

He was at the observation post.

Grenades hit it.

One hurt Pitts.

Others were killed.

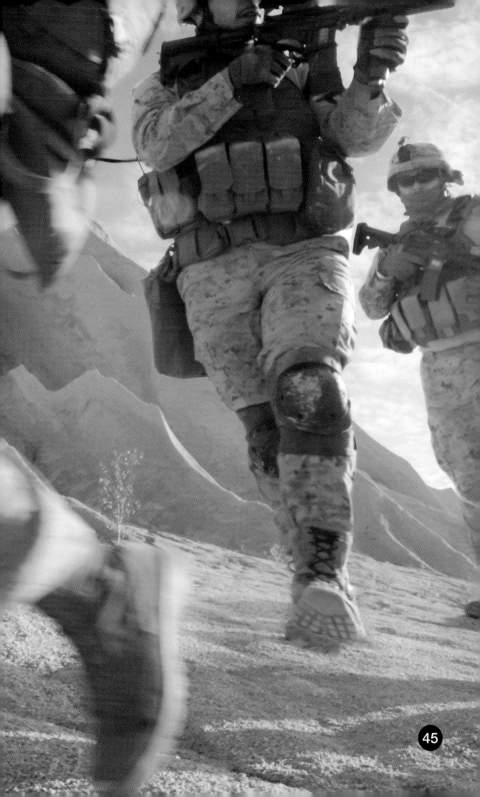

Pitts bled.

But he still fought.

Grenades were nearby.

He grabbed them.

Pitts pulled the pins.

He held the grenades.

They were about to blow.

Then he threw them.

The enemy could not get away.

Grenades blew right away.

Pitts could not stand.

He was near death.

Still he fought.

Help finally got there.

Pitts stopped the enemy.

He saved the post.

Now he has a Medal of Honor.

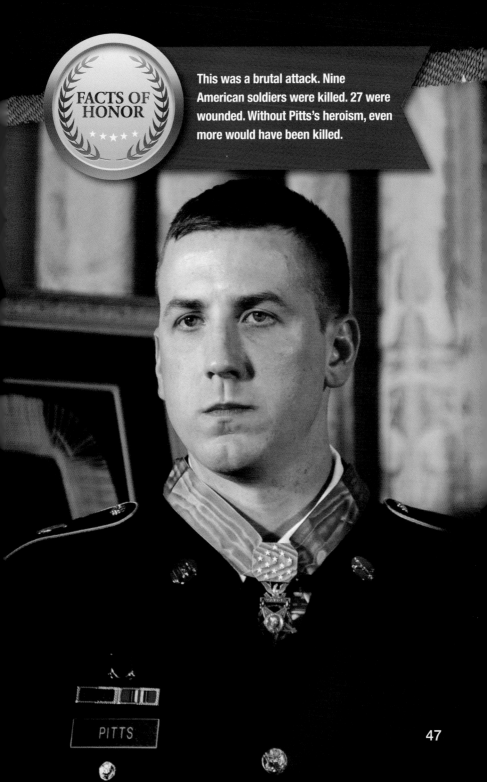

This was a brutal attack. Nine American soldiers were killed. 27 were wounded. Without Pitts's heroism, even more would have been killed.

PITTS

47

Chapter 10

HEROES

Soldiers answer a call.

It is the call of duty.

They serve their country.

Many come home.

Others are wounded.

They wear *scars*.

Some do not make it.

All soldiers know this.

But that does not stop them.

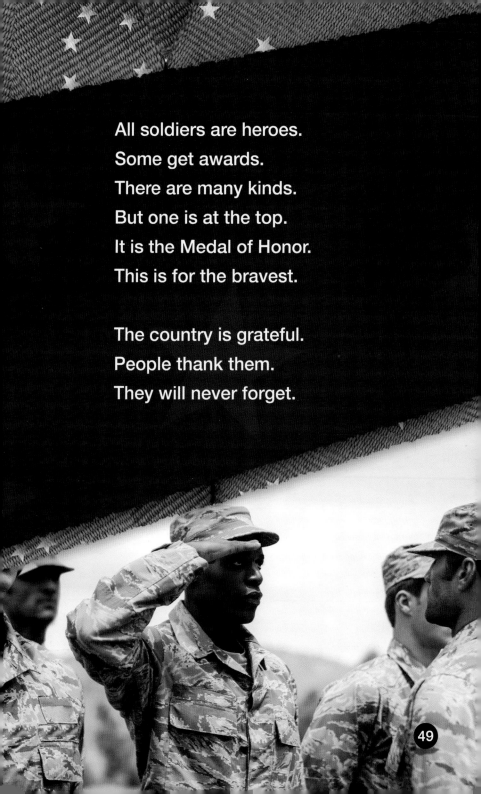

All soldiers are heroes.
Some get awards.
There are many kinds.
But one is at the top.
It is the Medal of Honor.
This is for the bravest.

The country is grateful.
People thank them.
They will never forget.

49

GLOSSARY

airstrip: land that is used as a runway for airplanes

bunker: a building that is used to keep soldiers and weapons safe during attacks; bunkers are often underground

chopper: a helicopter

duty: a job that a person is expected to do during certain hours

grenade: a small bomb that can be thrown or shot from a gun

gunner: a soldier who operates a large gun

hero: a person who is respected for being brave and doing great acts

honor: respect and recognition for a person

Medal of Honor: an award for valor in combat that is usually presented by the president in the name of Congress mortar: a cannon-like gun that is used in battle to fire shells; usually the gun fires at short range and low speed

patrol: going through an area to make sure it is safe

rights: privileges that belong to people and are protected by the law

scar: a mark left on the body after a wound heals

shell: a ball of metal that is full of explosive material from a mortar or other gun

soldier: a person who serves in the military

tank: a military vehicle that is covered with heavy armor

Underground Railroad: a network of safe houses and secret routes that helped slaves escape to freedom

Union: the Northern United States during the Civil War

valor: great bravery in the face of danger

wounded: hurt or injured

TAKE A LOOK INSIDE

TUSKEGEE AIRMEN

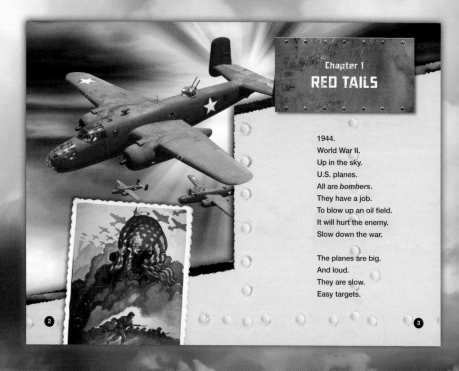

Chapter 1
RED TAILS

1944.
World War II.
Up in the sky.
U.S. planes.
All are *bombers*.
They have a job.
To blow up an oil field.
It will hurt the enemy.
Slow down the war.

The planes are big.
And loud.
They are slow.
Easy targets.

One man would not give up.
Yancey Williams.
He was black.
And a pilot.
He had a goal.
To join the U.S. Army Air Corps.
He passed the tests.
The Army still said no.
He went to court.
Fought for his *rights*.
It worked.

Chapter 5
THE EXPERIMENT

The Army changed its rules.
It did not want a court fight.
So it made a new unit.
The 99th Pursuit *Squadron*.
A group of planes.
Flown by blacks.
Williams saw this as a win.
He joined the unit.

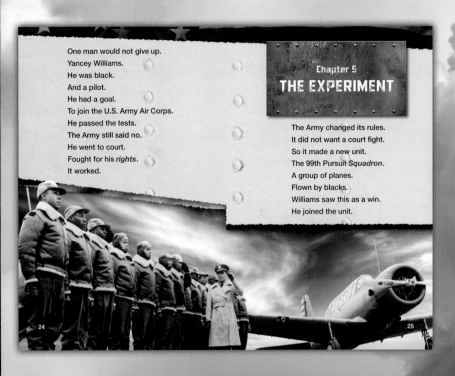

March 7, 1942.
A big day at Tuskegee.
The first class earned its wings.
Five men.
All ready to fly.

Who would lead them?
Benjamin O. Davis Jr.
He went to the U.S. Military Academy.
All the other *cadets* were white.
They did not talk to him.
But he stayed.
Studied hard.
And *graduated*.

Davis became an officer.
The Army chose him.
He would lead the 99th.
He had one goal.
"To lead this squadron to victory."

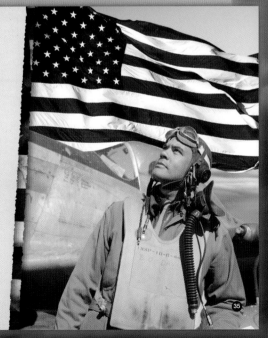

red rhino
books®

NONFICTION

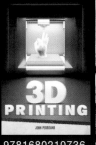
9781680210736

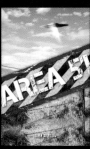
9781680210316

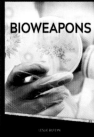
9781680210729

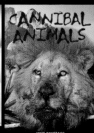
9781680210484

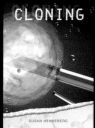
9781680210347

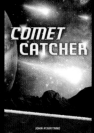
9781680210477

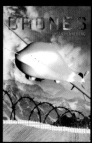
9781680210293

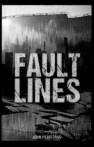
9781680210538

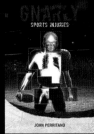
9781680210712

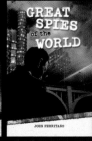
9781680210491

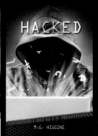
9781680210378

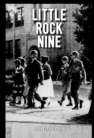
9781680210552

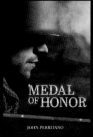
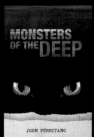
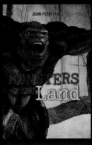
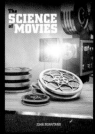
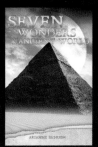
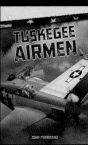
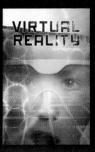
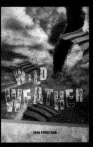
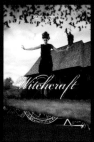
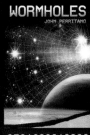